CONTENTS

EXAMINING THE CHILDREN'S GRADUATE MEDICAL EDUCATION PROGRAM

TUESDAY, MAY 9, 2006

HOUSE OF REPRESENTATIVES,
COMMITTEE ON ENERGY AND COMMERCE,
SUBCOMMITTEE ON HEALTH,
Washington, DC.

The subcommittee met, pursuant to notice, at 3:00 p.m., in Room 2322 of the Rayburn House Office Building, Hon. Nathan Deal (chairman of the subcommittee) presiding.

Present: Representatives Deal, Hall, Burgess, Brown, Waxman, Pallone, Capps, and Baldwin.

Staff Present: Randy Pate, Counsel; Katherine Martin, Professional Staff Member; Chad Grant, Legislative Clerk; John Ford, Minority Counsel; and Jessica McNiece, Minority Research Assistant.

MR. DEAL. The committee will come to order. The Chair recognizes himself for an opening statement.

I'm proud to say that we have three expert witnesses who are appearing before us this afternoon, who will help us examine the issues related to the reauthorization of enabling legislation for the Children's Hospital Graduate Medical Education Program.

Children's hospitals are an important part of our country's healthcare delivery system. They help improve by health outcomes by providing a unique set of specialized healthcare services and treatment options for children. As many of you know, this subcommittee has exclusive jurisdiction over the CHGME program, and we are committed to being good stewards of the program.

In all of my years of public service, I have never seen a perfect government program, and the CHGME program is certainly no exception to that rule. I firmly believe, however, that it is possible to improve the efficiency and the effectiveness of the program. To this end, I am particularly interested to hear from our witness from the Health Resources Service Administration about the Administration's proposals to reform the way in which funding is allocated under the program, and I am interested to hear the reaction to those proposals from our two children's hospital CEOs.

As we move forward with this reauthorization opportunity, it is my sincere hope that we can improve the outcomes of the CHGME program for the benefit of the children that these institutions serve.

At this time, I would like to ask unanimous consent that all members be able to submit statements and questions for the record, and without objection, it is so ordered.

[The prepared statement of Hon. Nathan Deal follows:]

PREPARED STATEMENT OF THE HON. NATHAN DEAL, CHAIRMAN, SUBCOMMITTEE ON HEALTH

The Committee will come to order, and the Chair recognizes himself for an opening statement.

I am proud to say that we have three expert witnesses appearing before us this afternoon that will help us examine the issues related to the reauthorization of enabling legislation for the Children's Hospital Graduate Medical Education Program.

Children's Hospitals are an important part of our country's health care delivery system. They improve health outcomes by providing a unique set of specialized health care services and treatment options for children. As many of you know, this Subcommittee has exclusive jurisdiction over the CHGME program, and we are committed to being good stewards of this program.

In all my years of public services, I have never seen a perfect government program, and the CHGME program is no exception. I firmly believe that it is possible to improve the efficiency and effectiveness of this program. To this end, I am particularly interested to hear from our witness from the Health Resources Service Administration about the Administration's proposals to reform the way in which funding is allocated under this program. And I am interested to hear the reaction to these proposals from our two Children's Hospital CEO's.

As we move forward with this reauthorization opportunity, it is my sincere hope that we can improve the outcomes of CHGME program for the benefit of the children that these institutions serve.

At this time, I would also like to ask for Unanimous Consent that all Committee Members be able to submit statements and questions for the record.

I now recognize the Ranking Member of the Subcommittee, Mr. Brown from Ohio, for five minutes for his opening statement.

MR. DEAL. I am now pleased to recognize the Ranking Member of the subcommittee, Mr. Brown from Ohio, for his opening statement.

MR. BROWN. Thank you, Mr. Chairman. Thank you to our witnesses, all three of you, for joining us this afternoon.

I particularly want to thank Bill Considine, the CEO of Akron Children's Hospital. I think he is the longest reigning CEO of any children's hospital in the country now, despite his youthful appearance. And Bill and several pediatricians at Akron General taught me about this issue many years ago, before anybody in this Congress knew about it, and talked about the impending problem, as managed care squeezed children's hospitals and all hospitals in their funding mechanisms, and what that meant to GME, and the funding of pediatric training, especially those pediatric specialists, many of whom are trained, some of the best are trained in our freestanding children's hospitals and other children's hospitals around the country.

In 1999, then Chairman Bilirakis and I introduced the legislation that established this program. Last year, Nancy Johnson and I introduced the pending reauthorization program. Each year, many of us, including on this committee, Mr. Waxman and Mr. Stupak, and I believe Ms. Capps and Ms. Baldwin also, gathered signatures in support of an ample appropriation for children's GME funding. This year, 218 members, a majority of this chamber, signed on.

Clearly, this program enjoys significant support in the House. It is the same in the Senate. In fact, they have already passed the reauthorization legislation. Now, it is our turn. There is solid logic behind the support this program enjoys. Historically, both Medicaid and most State Medicaid programs have provided funding for graduate medical education. Unfortunately, the Medicaid funding has never been sufficient. It has never even been consistent across different States, and now it is withering away as States cut their Medicaid budgets and contract with managed care plans unwilling to foot any of the GME bill.

Texas recently eliminated its Medicaid GME program. Other States will likely follow suit. Medicare has always been the larger of the two payers. It is a funding source upon which hospitals depend, except that is, for children's hospitals, especially those freestanding. My recollection is that Akron Children's, for instance, they have a burn unit which brings in some Medicare GME funding, and they get in-stage rail funding, as other Medicare GME programs do around the country, that brings money to children's hospitals. But other than that, that is about it.

Children's hospitals can't rely on Medicare GME funding because they don't have access to it. Under-investing in pediatric medicine makes no sense. We protect our children. We nurture our children. Why should we finance our way toward a healthcare system that shortchanges them? The answer is we shouldn't and we wouldn't.

The Children's GME program fills in the funding gap to provide public financing of GME, regardless of whether a hospital focuses on children or attends to the broader population. OMB has raised some concerns about children's GME, but it is almost as if they had a quota of concerns to fill, so they filled them. They talk about program accountability, but children's GME functions much the same as the regular GME program. Why is the children's program the target? Both programs could benefit from a better auditing process, and that process is going into place for the children's GME program. So, what is the problem again?

OMB also noted that children's hospitals receive Medicare GME. So do other hospitals, to the extent that--I am sorry, Medicaid GMEs. So do other hospitals, to the extent that Medicaid GME funding is still available. So, what actually is the point of OMB's finding? And OMB discusses the financial outlook for children's hospitals, both those freestanding, like Children's in Akron, or like Rainbow in Cleveland, it is affiliated with a larger hospital. It doesn't, though, discuss the financial outlook for other hospitals. That is because GME funding isn't linked to hospital finances. It is linked to the public's desire for well-trained health professionals. If children's hospitals are doing well, I would hope that is reflecting the availability, the quality, and the sophistication of the healthcare they provide. But GME is a public priority. That is true regardless of a hospital's year-to-year financial footing.

The President's budget proposes cutting the children's GME program by 66 percent. I propose that we invest where we need to invest before we drain the Federal budget into yet another round of billionaire tax cuts, something that my friends in this body want to do again. We want our children to thrive. We want sick children to get well. We want children with disabilities to fulfill their dreams. We can't do something for nothing.

Let us reauthorize children's GME. Let us fund it sufficiently, and let us resolve not to hurt kids as we choose. Do we give tax cuts to the wealthiest people in this country, or do we fund GME for children? It is a pretty simple choice.

Thank you, Mr. Chairman.

MR. DEAL. I recognize my friend from Texas, Mr. Hall, for an opening statement.

MR. HALL. Mr. Chairman, thank you.

You and the Ranking Member have done a very good job of laying it out, so I can be a little more brief. I am really pleased that you are having this hearing today on an issue that is very important, not just to any particular part of the Nation, but to all parts of the Nation.

Since 1999, the Graduate Medical Education funding has helped children's hospitals across the Nation reach a level of parity with other teaching hospitals. This program was established by Congress in recognition of an unfair disparity between medical education funding in adult versus children's hospitals, because children's hospitals do not treat Medicare patients and receive a GME pass-through from that program.

We have all heard, and we are likely to hear more today, about the growing shortage of qualified pediatric specialists, whether training in the pediatric field or researchers or whatever, the work of the children's hospitals in preparing doctors to further qualify pediatric healthcare is immeasurable.

So, I will just cut right through to it. Congress should continue to adequately fund and not cut graduate programs at these vital institutions, and I look forward to hearing from our panelists today, and I yield back the balance of my time.

MR. DEAL. I thank the gentleman. Ms. Capps, you are recognized for an opening statement.

MS. CAPPS. Thank you, Mr. Chairman. I thank you for holding this very important hearing today to highlight children's hospitals graduate medical education.

Children's GME programs are the backbone of training pediatricians, pediatric specialists, and pediatric researchers, and in the State from which Mr. Waxman and I come, California, we have seven children's hospitals that receive children's GME, who alone train hundreds of residents, nearly half of whom are trained in pediatric specialties. This is very vital to the care of our sick children.

Today, our country is experiencing a shortage of pediatric specialists. I think no one disagrees with that statement, and it is our children's hospitals, where they receive the training, the skill sets, to fill these positions. At the same time they are devoting resources to training new residents, they are also treating the Nation's sickest children, who are more often than not being covered by Medicaid. These are children suffering from cancer, children needing organ transplants, children needing heart surgery. The list goes on and on. Since the authorization of the children's GME program through this committee in 1999, we have enabled a response to the shortage of physicians able to treat children with life-threatening, chronic, or rare diseases.

Children's GME programs currently get less funding than other GME programs, a disparity that is current, but there has been, over the past few years, significant progress. It is, therefore, very astounding to me that this Administration has proposed such a severe reduction in funding, by two-thirds for these programs, just in one year. I am sure we will hear today the argument that it is due to budget constraints, but I think we need to look at the facts, and look at the real world. Training more doctors now, providing children's hospitals with better resources to treat and early identify their patients, many of whom are on Medicaid, is certainly going to translate into cost savings later. We will be able to better diagnose and better treat children early on, before they become sicker, more disabled, more costly to treat.

So, I look forward to hearing from our witnesses today, who represent two of our Nation's children's hospitals, about the successes that children's GME has provided in the field. More importantly, I want to learn why the Administration has chosen to jeopardize, practically eliminate this program.

I yield back.

MR. DEAL. I thank the gentlelady. Mr. Waxman, you are recognized for an opening statement.

MR. WAXMAN. Mr. Chairman, I am pleased this subcommittee is holding a hearing today to examine the success of the children's hospital GME program, because a success it has been.

As you know, whether by design or accident, this country supports its graduate medical education through payments made as part of the Medicare program. Generally, that has worked well and achieved its goal, but one critical set of hospitals was essentially left out, and that was children's hospitals. Yet these institutions have a critical role in training physicians, particularly pediatric and pediatric specialty residents in doing research and in serving as centers of excellence for serving children.

We attempted to correct that problem when we passed a program in the Public Health Service Act to provide critical GME support to children's hospitals. That program has enjoyed strong bipartisan support from the beginning, and has made a critical contribution to the training of physicians, the care of our children, and the financial health of children's hospitals, and that is why it is particularly distressing to me that the Administration has shown so little support for this program, keeps trying to cut its funding, and now is attempting to revise the legislative authority as well.

They want to impose a principle of directing funds only to children's hospitals that are in critical financial circumstances, yet I note that they are not similarly concerned about how the Medicare program support operates. They recognize that there, that the support must be provided to all hospitals with GME costs. Why should children's hospitals, which play such a critical role in our society, be treated less generously?

I have a wonderful children's hospital that serves the children in my district and greater Los Angeles. While nearly half of its patients are Medicaid beneficiaries, it is an important source of care for all children. It is a valued resource in the community, and I think this is typical of the view of children's hospitals around the Nation. I hope that after this hearing today, we will reaffirm our support for the children's hospitals GME program and for the wonderful institutions that receive funding from it.

Thank you.

MR. DEAL. I thank the gentleman. Ms. Baldwin, you are recognized for an opening statement.

MS. BALDWIN. Thank you, Mr. Chairman, and I also want to thank the witnesses who are joining us today.

Like many of my colleagues, I am a proud supporter of the Children's Hospital GME Program. Children's hospitals play a vital role in training the doctors who will care for our Nation's children in the future, and it is important that we support them in this critical endeavor.

The program has had a remarkable success in both stemming reductions in the number of pediatric residents, and also, in helping to provide stability for children's hospitals. I know that the Wisconsin Children's Hospital in Milwaukee has directly benefited from the Children's Hospital GME program, and that the University of Wisconsin's Children's Hospital in my district, although not eligible for Children's Hospital GME payments, has also benefited from the program, because the program has helped to train pediatricians who bring their expertise to the UW.

I am sorry to note that this program expired at the end of fiscal year 2005. A program like this, that has such strong bipartisan support deserves better. And we all know what happens to programs when their authorizations are allowed to lapse. Slowly, but surely, we see their appropriations levels drop. In fiscal year 2005, the Children's Hospital GME program received $300 million. That fell to $297 million in fiscal year 2006, and the President, in his fiscal year 2007 budget, proposed drastically cutting the funding to $99 million. Who knows what will happen if the House ever passes a fiscal year 2007 budget resolution? But one thing I do know is that this program provides valuable services, and it deserves to be fully funded.

I would also like to spend a brief moment reflecting on the environment in which children's hospitals operate. They are major providers of services to low-income children. In fact, more than 47 percent of their days of care, on average, are for children covered by Medicaid. As we see pressure on the Medicaid budget continue, and as the majority in Congress weakens the program as was done recently during the last year's budget reconciliation process, it becomes even more vital that we support children's hospitals GME.

So, I am happy that the committee has decided to take up this issue, and I look forward to working with my fellow Members on moving forward with a reauthorization bill. And thank you, Mr. Chairman. I yield back my remaining time.

MR. DEAL. I thank the gentlelady. Mr. Pallone, you are recognized for an opening statement.

MR. PALLONE. Thank you, Mr. Chairman. I want to, in some ways, repeat what some of my colleagues said, and also add to it, if I can.

I do have a number of children's hospitals in my district, and of course, the one that immediately comes to mind is the one in New Brunswick, which is increasingly the health center for the State of New Jersey. And listening to what my colleague, Ms. Baldwin, said in particular applies to New Brunswick, where we have a large Medicaid population. Today, in fact, there was much made in the media in New Jersey about the fact that the Governor, because of budget shortfalls, is having a hard time even keeping up with the family care program, because of the SCHIP program, I should say, as we know it here, because of Federal budget cuts, as well as the State budget crisis. So, all the things that my colleague from Wisconsin mentioned about the impact on children's healthcare is, I think, even more magnified in my home State of New Jersey these days, and particularly, in New Brunswick, which is a center, because of their children's hospital.

The other thing I have to tell you is that you know, I have a sort of special reason to be opposed to what the President is proposing here with these cuts in the children's hospital GME program. First of all, because my next door neighbor is a pediatrician and has practically raised my three children when I am not there, and he is constantly pointing out to me, as my wife does constantly, about how we neglect children that the Federal government and the Congress, because they are not voters, essentially, are neglected.

And it is pretty sad to think that, hospitals are able to rely, because they have a large Medicare and senior population, and because seniors vote, that we link formulas to them, but then at the same time, because the children's hospital doesn't have the Medicare population, that they, you know, that they have a funding shortfall. So, this GME program was designed essentially to make up for the fact that there are a lot of children's hospitals that don't have this Medicare population and therefore have the funding shortfalls.

For us to now turn around and say, as the President does, that we are going to change this, and make those cuts, I think directly goes back to the fact that children are not represented, that children are not viewed positively by politicians, and I think that, you know, those of us who feel strongly that it shouldn't be that way need to speak out against these types of cuts.

The other thing I would point out is that this subcommittee and this committee in general, has been very much trying to promote research in children's diseases. I remember Mr. Waxman, Mr. Brown, on many occasions pointing out that a lot of times, when we come to drugs in particular, but other things as well, that we need to do more research on the impact on children, but that is not done, and I know that that is, in fact, done in New Brunswick at the children's hospital. I know that a lot of these hospitals are doing a lot of research that directly relates to how drugs and other things impact children.

So, this is not the time to cut this. We need these residents. We need the research, and we certainly shouldn't be discriminating against children, which this children's hospital GME program was designed to overcome.

So, I think it is very important to have this hearing today, and I appreciate the fact that we are paying attention to it on both sides of the aisle.

Thank you, Mr. Chairman.

[Additional statements for the record follow:]

PREPARED STATEMENT OF THE HON. JOE BARTON, CHAIRMAN, COMMITTEE ON ENERGY AND COMMERCE

Thank you Chairman Deal for holding this hearing on the Children's Hospital Graduate Medical Education program, commonly referred to as CHGME.

First established in 1999, the program was designed to better balance the levels of federal funding for adult teaching hospitals and children's teaching hospitals. The program helps children's hospitals which do not receive a significant amount of federal dollars for their residential training programs because of low volumes of Medicare patients. The nation's sixty teaching children's hospitals are responsible for the education of nearly one out of three pediatricians and half of all pediatric specialists.

The Administration has proposed several reforms to the program in its FY 2007 Budget. Specifically, the President wants the program to prioritize payments to hospitals that demonstrate the greatest financial need; that treat the largest number of uninsured patients; and that train the greatest number of physicians.

This Committee has been very active in looking at all programs within our jurisdiction, with particular emphasis paid to those with expiring authorizations. It is our responsibility to recipients of federal dollars and, of course, to the taxpayers to ensure each program is structured to achieve optimal efficiency and effectiveness. We should examine proposed reforms with these goals always in mind.

I hope this hearing provides an opportunity to examine issues related to reauthorization of the program and the potential need for structural reform. I expect this Committee to consider reauthorization legislation in the near future. Thank you again Chairman Deal for holding today's hearing and welcome to our witnesses.

PREPARED STATEMENT OF THE HON. BARBARA CUBIN, A REPRESENTATIVE IN CONGRESS FROM THE STATE OF WYOMING

Thank you Mr. Chairman.

Today we have an opportunity to take a close look at the impact of Children's Hospitals Graduate Medical Education (GME) Program on communities across the nation. First authorized in 1999, the program has proved to be of tremendous help in supporting graduate medical education training at Children's hospitals.

Congress again amended and reviewed this program in 2004, and over the past three fiscal years has approved a level funding allocation of $303 million. In Fiscal Year 2007, the Administration has proposed to reduce the program to $99 million, a drastic reduction that gives me pause considering the impact of the program on the State of Wyoming.

While the State of Wyoming is without a children's hospital, the Children's Hospital in Denver, CO serves thousands of Wyoming patients in need of care. The facility is also a valuable training resource in the region. There are at least sixteen physicians currently practicing in Wyoming who trained at the hospital. Other residents complete rural rotations, providing care to communities throughout the state. We have a shortage of health professionals in the state and we need all the providers that we can muster.

I hope our Health Resources and Services Administration panelist will be able to shed some light on why the Administration feels the GME Program cut is necessary. I understand the merits of trying to improve accountability in the program and ensure that federal aid is appropriately targeted, especially given the budget crunch we are facing. Even as we tighten our fiscal belts, however, we must be careful not to throw the baby out with the bath water.

PREPARED STATEMENT OF THE HON. ANNA ESHOO, A REPRESENTATIVE IN CONGRESS FROM THE STATE OF CALIFORNIA

Thank you, Mr. Chairman for holding this important hearing.

As an original cosponsor of the Children's Hospitals Education Equity and Research (CHEER) Act, I hope we can move on a reauthorization of the Children's Hospital Graduate Medical Education program soon.

I'm proud to represent one of the leading children's hospitals in the country – Lucile Packard Children's Hospital.

The work that's been pioneered at Packard has benefited not only patients from throughout the country, it has also benefited patients at other hospitals through techniques which have been developed at Packard by the personnel trained there.

I'm sure every children's hospital which receives funding under the CHGME program can make a similar claim.

CHGME hospitals train 30% of all pediatricians, half of all pediatric subspecialists, and the majority of pediatric researchers in our country.

In California alone, CHGME program funds are used by 7 children's hospitals to train 652 full-time residents annually, with 318 trained in a pediatric subspecialty.

These hospitals treat the most difficult cases, often children from families who do not have the resources to pay for treatment on their own. In California, more than half of the children cared for are Medicaid eligible.

With such a record, it's difficult for me to comprehend why the Administration proposes to cut the CHGME program from its current appropriated level of $297 million to $99 million in fiscal year 2007, and scale back the program in the next reauthorization.

No one in the health care community supports this proposal, and beyond the desire to cut spending, there can be no justifications for such a draconian cut.

The Administration has made this proposal solely for the Children's Hospital GME program, not for the Medicare GME program, even though the Medicare GME program reimburses at a higher rate.

Mr. Chairman, I hope our Committee will recognize how shortsighted the Administration's proposal is and then will move forward in a bipartisan manner to reauthorize the CHGME program as the Senate has already done.

PREPARED STATEMENT OF THE HON. GENE GREEN, A REPRESENTATIVE IN CONGRESS FROM THE STATE OF TEXAS

Thank you, Mr. Chairman, for holding this hearing on the Children's Hospital Graduate Medical Education Program (CHGME). We in Congress established this program nearly seven years ago in recognition of the federal support needed for training activities at our children's teaching hospitals. In other hospital settings, training dollars needed for residents are funded, in part, through Medicare's graduate medical education program. With relatively few Medicare patients being served at children's hospitals, however, children's teaching hospitals cannot fully benefit from Medicare's graduate medical education program. CHGME was established to help alleviate the inequity faced by children's hospitals with respect to the training of their residents.

Since its inception in 1999, the CHGME program has achieved tremendous success and enabled our children's teaching hospitals to address reductions in the number of pediatric residents. With this funding, children's teaching hospitals – such as Texas Children's Hospital in my hometown of Houston – have been able to keep their residency programs alive and ensure that the pediatricians treating our children and our grandchildren are trained at the best facilities in the country.

It's no surprise that the same children's teaching hospitals receiving CHGME funds provide the ideal training grounds for pediatric residents. These hospitals house the nation's leading pediatric research institutions and provide residents with experience in treating the whole gamut of childhood health care problems, from routine immunizations to pediatric trauma care and pediatric oncology.

Continued CHGME funding is critical if our children's hospitals are going to continue providing quality care to low-income children, as well as children whose families have private health insurance. Nearly fifty percent of care delivered at our children's hospitals nationwide is provided to Medicaid beneficiaries, and CHGME payments help cover the gap created by a Medicaid reimbursement policy that covers only 80 percent of care delivered to Medicaid patients.

The CHGME program provides children's teaching hospitals with real funding, without which their residency programs would face severe financial strain. Texas Children's Hospital in Houston is one of the top children's hospitals in the country and received nearly $11 million last year in CHGME payments. Even with this funding, Texas Children's absorbed an additional $11.5 million in unreimbursed costs associated with their training of pediatric residents.

We want our pediatricians trained at quality hospitals like Texas Children's, where they can put their skills to use on a diverse set of patients with varying diagnoses. Through this type of education and training, pediatric residents can leave children's teaching hospitals and travel to all corners of the country armed with the experience to effectively treat the young patients in their community. CHGME makes this possible, and I join my colleagues in supporting the reauthorization of this important program.

PREPARED STATEMENT OF THE HON. GEORGE RADANOVICH, A REPRESENTATIVE IN CONGRESS FROM THE STATE OF CALIFORNIA

I would first like to thank the Chairman for his leadership on this issue, and for calling this important hearing looking into the reauthorization of the Children's Hospital Graduate Medical Education Program. This is an extremely important program that has consistently proven well worth the investment we make, and I am very glad to see this committee addressing the needs of Children's Graduate Hospital Medical Education.

When Congress first authorized $285 million in 1999 for this program, we were addressing the unintended inequity created by government financing of graduate medical education. Since that time, children's hospitals have utilized these funds to increase the numbers of residents they train, types of training programs they provide, and quality of the training offered. This has all been done without having to compromise clinical care or research.

Children's hospitals continually strive to see that every child has access to high quality, cost efficient care. In doing so, they can save taxpayers money by providing the preventive care necessary to ensure that many problems are detected, addressed and treated before they become much more expensive emergencies and chronic problems in the future. I have had the pleasure of personally visiting some of the fine safety net children's care providers around my district in California, and I can assure you first hand that the work done in these children's hospitals is literally saving lives. Through the funds provided by the Children's Hospital Graduate Medical Education Program, California hospitals have been able to increase their quality and availability of care, even at a time when the country is experiencing a shortage of pediatric specialists.

However, to allow them to continue to do their work we must ensure that there the funds are available to help cover the costs incurred at children's hospitals for the training of pediatricians and children's healthcare specialists.

Mr. Chairman, I am a proud cosponsor of HR 1246, the "Children's Hospital Equity Education and Research", also known as the "CHEER", Act. I thank the gentlelady from Connecticut, Mrs. Johnson, for introducing this important legislation. I understand and agree with the Administration that we need to try to reduce spending where possible, but I do not think this is the appropriate area to do so and that the funding request in the President's Budget Proposal of $99 million for this year – a $198 million reduction from last year – is inadequate.

The best way to utilize limited healthcare funds is to ensure that we provide them to programs that will efficiently use the money to produce results. I don't believe there is any question that funding for children's graduate medical education produces results.
I thank the Chairman again for his leadership, thank our witnesses for being here today to share their expertise, and look forward to a productive and informative hearing on how we can best support Children's Hospital Graduate Medical Education Programs.

MR. DEAL. Well, that will conclude our opening statements. We are pleased to have our first panelist, Ms. Kerry Nesseler, who is the Associate Administrator for Health Professions of the Health Resources and Services Administration of the U.S. Department of Health and Human Services.

Ms. Nesseler, we are pleased to have you here. I would remind you that your printed testimony is already a part of the record, as I would advise the other witnesses. We already have your printed testimony. It has been available to the panel. We appreciate that.

Ms. Nesseler, we are pleased to have you here, and we will recognize you for your opening statement.

MS. NESSELER. Thank you, Mr. Chairman. I am pleased to be here also. I request permission to submit to the record my entire written statement.

MR. DEAL. Yes, it is already a part of the record.

STATEMENT OF KERRY NESSELER, ASSOCIATE ADMINISTRATOR, BUREAU OF HEALTH PROFESSIONS, HEALTH RESOURCES AND SERVICES ADMINISTRATION, U.S. DEPARTMENT OF HEALTH AND HUMAN SERVICES

MS. NESSELER. Mr. Chairman, members of the subcommittee, thank you for the opportunity to meet with you today on behalf of the Health

Resources Services Administration, HRSA, to discuss the Children's Hospitals Graduate Medical Education Program.

The Children's Hospitals Graduate Medical Education Program was authorized by the Healthcare Research and Quality Act of 1999. The program was amended by the Children's Healthcare Act of 2000, and was further amended in 2004. Its purpose is to support graduate medical education training in freestanding children's teaching hospitals. And payments are made to these hospitals to enhance their financial viability.

The Children's Hospitals Graduate Medical Education Program addresses the need for funds beyond patient revenues to support the broad teaching mission of freestanding children's teaching hospitals, which includes conducting biomedical research, training health professionals, providing rare and highly specialized clinical services, innovative clinical care, and providing care to the poor and the underserved. Teaching hospitals have higher costs than other hospitals because of the special services they provide.

The program currently disburses Direct Medical Education and Indirect Medical Education payments to eligible and participating children's hospitals. Based on Congressional mandate, one third of the total appropriated funds are disbursed for direct medical education, and the remaining two thirds are disbursed for indirect medical education. A Children's Hospital's GME Payment Program's DME allocation, and those are costs associated with training the residents, is based on the national updated per resident amounts, as defined by Section 340E(c)(2) of the Public Health Service Act, and the 3-years rolling average of weighted full-time equivalent medical resident counts as determined under Section 1886(h)(4) of the Social Security Act. A Children's Hospitals GME Payment Program's IME, indirect medical education, payments are the payments associated with adjustments for the cost of direct patient care. Currently, IME payments are determined by: one, participating children's hospitals numbers of discharge; two, the severity of illness of the patient population, using a case mix index; and three, the teaching intensity factor, as captured by the resident-to-bed ratio.

In fiscal year '05, the Children's Hospitals GME supported 61 freestanding children's hospitals and the training of about 4,892 medical residents on and offsite. The program, as currently implemented, is in need of change. The President's fiscal year 2007 budget requests $99 million to support the mission of children's teaching hospitals.

To support this budget request, the Administration is proposing legislative reform of this program, specifically with the IME payments. The DME, direct medical education payments, which are associated with training of medical residents, will remain the same. The President's budget proposes ensuring access to care by supporting children's hospitals based on: one, their financial status; and two, the children's hospitals who continue to care for those children who are underinsured or uninsured. Participating children's hospitals would be required to account for the use of these Federal funds, and have clear, standardized performance requirements, such as the effect of program funds on improvement in patient care.

Under this new proposal, we emphasize that payments will focus on those children's hospitals with one, the greatest financial need; two, that treat the largest number of uninsured patients; and three, that train the greatest number of physicians.

The proposed legislative reform is designed to better target limited Federal resources where they are needed most. Federal support would be provided to ensure that the pediatricians first will continue to receive the best training possible, with the objective of achieving improvements in patient care outcomes. Reporting requirements on the use of funds will demonstrate the results achieved by freestanding children's hospitals in performing their three-pronged mission, as teaching hospitals, safety-net providers, and providers of quality care for children.

Under this proposal, Federal support for direct medical education, which is the training of physicians, will continue to depend on the number of full-time equivalent residents trained. The President's new formulation will replace the current indirect medical education payment formula, which currently accounts for the teaching intensity, which is using residents-to-bed ratio; the number of patient discharges; and the severity of illness of the inpatient population. Federal support will be distributed based again on the volume of uncompensated care provided by the institution and two, the financial status of the hospitals.

The impact of the proposal is to target the funds to help children's hospitals caring for the poor and the underserved, and help the children's hospitals that are in the greatest financial need.

Thank you for this opportunity to discuss the Administration's principles for the legislative reform of the Children's Hospitals Graduate Medical Education Program. We look forward to working with this subcommittee on this proposal.

[The prepared statement of Kerry Nesseler follows:]

PREPARED STATEMENT OF KERRY NESSELER, R.N., M.S., ASSOCIATE ADMINISTRATOR, BUREAU OF HEALTH PROFESSIONS, HEALTH RESOURCES AND SERVICES ADMINISTRATION, U.S. DEPARTMENT OF HEALTH AND HUMAN SERVICES

Mr. Chairman, Members of the Subcommittee, thank you for the opportunity to meet with you today on behalf of the Health Resources and Services Administration (HRSA) to discuss the Children's Hospitals Graduate Medical Education Program.

<u>Background</u>

The Children's Hospitals Graduate Medical Education Program was authorized by the Healthcare Research and Quality Act of 1999. The program was amended by the Children's Health Act of 2000 and was further amended in 2004. Its purpose is to support graduate medical education (GME) training in freestanding children's teaching hospitals. Payments are made to these hospitals to enhance their financial viability.

The Children's Hospitals GME Program addresses the need for funds beyond patient revenues to support the broad teaching mission of freestanding children's teaching hospitals, which includes conducting biomedical research, training health professionals, providing rare and highly specialized clinical services and innovative clinical care, and providing care to the poor and the underserved. Teaching hospitals have higher costs than other hospitals because of the special services they provide.

Implementation

The program currently disburses Direct Medical Education (DME) and Indirect Medical Education (IME) payments to eligible and participating children's hospitals. Based on Congressional mandate, one-third of total appropriated funds are disbursed for DME and the remaining two-thirds are disbursed for IME. A Children's Hospitals GME Payment Program's participating hospital's DME payment allocation is based on the national updated per-resident amounts as defined by §340E(c)(2) of the Public Health Service Act and the three years rolling average of weighted full time equivalent medical resident counts as determined under §1886(h)(4) of the Social Security Act. A Children's Hospitals GME Payment Program's IME payments are determined by a participating children's hospital's capacity to treat patients (number of discharges), severity of illness of the patients population (using a case mix index), and the teaching intensity factor as captured by the intern-resident to bed ratio.

In fiscal year (FY) 2004, the Children's Hospitals GME supported 61 freestanding children's hospitals and the training of 4,892 medical residents on and off site. The financial support for the training of medical residents is based on a three-year rolling average of weighted and unweighted full time equivalent residents, number of discharges, number of available beds, and a case mix index. The program as currently implemented is in need of change.

Proposal

The President's FY 2007 Budget requests $99 million to support the mission of children's teaching hospitals, which includes training medical residents, ensuring access to care by supporting children's hospitals based on their financial status, and encouraging the children's hospitals to continue caring for those children who are underinsured or uninsured.

To support this Budget Request, the Administration is proposing legislative reform of this program. The proposal will address specific needs of children's hospitals in the nation. Under this new program, funds will be distributed based on the financial status of freestanding children's hospitals, their uncompensated care caseload, and the number of full time equivalent medical residents (including interns and fellows) in training. The payment formula will weight financial status, uncompensated care, and number of full time equivalent medical residents (interns and fellows) in training. Participating children's hospitals would be required to account for the use of these Federal funds, and have clear, standardized performance requirements, such as the effect of program funds on improvements in patient care. Under this new proposal, we emphasize that payments will focus on those children's hospitals with the greatest financial need that treat the largest number of uninsured patients and train the greatest number of physicians.

Rationale

The proposed legislative reform is designed to better target limited Federal resources where they are needed most. Federal support will be provided to ensure that the pediatric workforce will continue to receive the best training possible with the objective of achieving improvement in patient care outcomes. Furthermore, Federal support will be provided to those freestanding children's hospitals with the greatest financial need, and Federal support will be provided to encourage teaching hospitals to continue providing quality patient care to those children who are without a source of payment or are underinsured. Reporting requirements on the use of funds will demonstrate the results achieved by freestanding children's hospitals in performing their three-pronged mission as teaching hospitals, safety net providers, and providers of quality care for children.

Impact

Under this proposal, Federal support for the training of physicians will continue to depend on the number of full time equivalent residents trained, the national average per resident amount adjusted for labor and non-labor share and geographic distances.

The impact and reasoning of the proposal is to target the funds to help children's hospitals caring for the poor and underserved, and help children's hospitals that are in the greatest financial need. This new formulation will replace the current Indirect Medical Education payment formula which accounts for teaching intensity (using the interns and residents to bed ratio), capacity for patient care (number of inpatient discharges), and severity of illness (case mix index) of the inpatient population. Federal support for uncompensated care will be distributed based on the volume of uncompensated care provided by the institution.

Conclusion

Thank you for the opportunity to discuss the Administration's principles for the legislative reform of the Children's Hospitals Graduate Medical Education Program. We look forward to working with this Subcommittee on this proposal.

MR. DEAL. Well, thank you.

You have heard the concerns that have been expressed in the opening statements on both sides here--

MS. NESSELER. Yes, sir.

MR. DEAL. --about the proposed reductions in funding of the payment program for graduate medical education--

MS. NESSELER. Yes, sir.

MR. DEAL. --in children's hospitals. Would you comment on what you think the impact of such a reduction in funding would actually be?

MS. NESSELER. Well, sir, currently the Administration is still proposing Federal support for this graduate medical education training at freestanding children's hospital.

The Administration is trying to align Federal support with the mission of teaching hospitals. Federal graduate medical education support for freestanding teaching hospitals comes from appropriated funds which are limited, while support for the adult teaching hospitals is provided through a Medicare trust fund. We believe the FY 2007 budget request of $99 million is good, strong funding for children's hospitals, and especially, if we focus on children's hospitals that need it the most, and do provide care to the most underserved populations.

MR. DEAL. You mentioned in your testimony that statute currently sets the ratio between the IME and the DME.

MS. NESSELER. Yes, sir.

MR. DEAL. Are you proposing that that formula be changed, as to the proportion? As I see the proposal, the DME would actually consume the entire $99 million, if we didn't do anything to change the formula allocations. Are you proposing changing the formula allocations?

MS. NESSELER. Yes, sir. Currently, as it stands, one-third goes to direct medical education, and two-thirds goes to indirect medical education. And we are looking at keeping the direct medical education formula mostly the same, but looking at about 40 percent for DME. And then, this second piece, which is about 60 percent, is again looking at the financial status, and the number of uncompensated care patients that they treat.

MR. DEAL. Being someone who comes from a rural area--

MS. NESSELER. Yes, sir.

MR. DEAL. --I am concerned about the lack of children's teaching hospitals in most rural areas. Does the Administration have any proposal with regard to children's hospitals in more rural areas that may not quite have the caseload to qualify for some of these funds?

MS. NESSELER. Currently, we do not. It is under discussion of how we will determine financial need, and how we will determine uncompensated care and the increased numbers of patients seen that are uninsured. That is under discussion at this point, but I do not have a formula.

MR. DEAL. This is a little bit of a complicated question, so I am going to read it, but--

MS. NESSELER. Yes, sir.

MR. DEAL. --it is an important piece of information we need to know. Medicare allows low Medicare utilization hospitals, such as children's hospitals, to file low-volume reports that do not contain all the cost information required for the full-cost report.

Do you believe your agency has sufficient information regarding the financial status of all the participating children's hospitals, bed count, patient volume, and other such data points, to effectively make changes to the program, or will you require some additional information and reporting on those items?

MS. NESSELER. We currently believe we get sufficient information. Yes, we do get cost reports from all of our 61 children's hospitals. Some are larger reports, depending on how much Medicare dollars they get; depending on how much chronic care that they provide, like dialysis; and that is how they receive their additional extra Medicare payments. But yes, we do feel we have sufficient cost reporting.

MR. DEAL. And from what other sources do children's teaching hospitals receive funding, and does this other source include GME funding?

MS. NESSELER. Other sources of funding are, again, a bit of Medicare dollars, if they are taking care of chronically ill children, such as dialysis patients, or severe heart problems. They receive funding from State Medicaid. They receive a lot of private dollars also, sir, in addition to the Federal dollars.

MR. DEAL. Many of them receive rather significant private contributions, I believe, do they not?

MS. NESSELER. Sir, I can get you an answer for the record. I don't have that exact number.

MR. DEAL. All right. It appears that the direct medical education dollars are allocated to hospitals on a per resident formula, and IME dollars are determined by a number of factors. Can you better explain to us how these dollars are currently distributed? Maybe you have already touched on that, but--

MS. NESSELER. Yes, I can. Currently, I guess about one-third of the dollars go for direct medical education, and that is literally the training of the physicians, which are mostly pediatricians and sub-specialists in pediatrics. That is for their salaries, for their stipends, so that goes for direct medical education, about a third of the dollars. Two-thirds of the dollars goes for indirect medical education. And that is a combination between the children's hospital capacity to treat patients, which is their number of discharges; the severity of the illnesses of the patient population, if you have a NICU, neonatal intensive care unit, or a burn center, there are more severe patients at that hospital, and that uses a case mix index. And also, the teaching intensity factor, as captured by the resident-to-bed ratio, or how many physicians for how many beds, if it is a higher or lower number. That is currently how it is, and that is two-thirds.

MR. DEAL. Mr. Brown, you are recognized for questions.

MR. BROWN. Thank you, Mr. Chairman. Thank you, Ms. Nesseler, for joining us.

MS. NESSELER. Thank you, sir.

MR. BROWN. And I appreciate your testimony.

I am trying to understand why the Administration wants to cut children's GME. I mean, this has been a battle really since the early part of this century. I mean, for the last five years, it has always been an issue with this Administration on GME.

There were a couple of hints in the OMB that, looking at this, there seemed to be a couple of hints in OMB's program assessment. From my understanding, what they were able to, and if you kind of read between the lines, they seem to say that the money that went to GME, and Akron Children's or Rainbow or Columbus Children's or whatever, that that money could be used for other things, and they weren't so sure the money was really going to what it was intended. But my understanding is the larger GME program works the same way. We don't tell the Boston and New York hospitals, or we don't tell any of the hospitals that generally address illness for the general population, we don't tell them specifically where their GME money goes, either. Is that the right assessment, generally?

MS. NESSELER. Sir, I am not as familiar with the CMS adult hospitals. I can tell you under the PART score, we did get a rating of adequate. And we really look at $99 million as a sufficient budget for children's hospitals GME. The PART score of adequate gave us two recommendations: to look more closely at auditing, and to do an objective evaluation study. Those are two, so according to us, this program has been very successful. We believe the $99 million is adequate if we are looking at the hospitals with the highest need. With the PART score of adequate, we have a little bit of work to do, but we feel as though we have done well with the program, sir.

MR. BROWN. But generally, GME to other hospitals goes without strings attached, correct? When GME funding goes to any large hospital that doesn't just focus on children, the money is--

MS. NESSELER. Correct, for adult hospitals.

MR. BROWN. Yeah, it is not connected to--we want to make sure we know where every penny that we are giving you goes, that this dollar goes to training of specialists, this dollar goes to salaries and equipment and training of new doctors, correct?

MS. NESSELER. Sir, I am not a witness to testify for CMS adult hospitals, and I could get some answers to the record for you, but I don't feel--

MR. BROWN. If you would. Okay. Shift to Medicaid for a minute. Medicaid provides funding in some States to hospitals in other States, as in Texas, and in others to follows. It doesn't. Children's hospitals, I believe, discuss that with me for a moment, what you see for the future, if these States, if States begin to cut back, as Texas is, cuts back its Medicaid funding for GME, what kind of impact will that have, in your mind?

MS. NESSELER. Currently, we are looking at hospitals with the greatest financial need, and that the $99 million is a sufficient budget to keep their services. That is all I can say, sir.

MR. BROWN. Okay. Thanks.

MS. NESSELER. Thank you.

MR. DEAL. Mr. Hall, you are recognized for questions.

MR. HALL. What is the source of a cut of that magnitude, $297 million, down to $99 million? They are cutting out $198 million.

MS. NESSELER. Yes, sir.

MR. HALL. What is the source of that? Whose decision was that?

MS. NESSELER. Sir, it is the President's '07 budget proposal to Congress.

MR. HALL. Well, who proposed that to him? Were you part of the group that proposed that to him?

MS. NESSELER. Sir, it comes from the President.

MR. HALL. And you really don't agree with it, do you, deep down in your heart?

MS. NESSELER. Sir, I am a maternal child health nurse, and I am very committed to maternal child health, which includes children's, and the President is committed, also, with $99 million, to treat children at children's hospitals, yes, sir.

MR. HALL. Well, I understand you almost have to be in that position, don't you?.

MS. NESSELER. Sir, I--

MR. HALL. You are representing the President, and you are doing the best you can do for the President. Right? And his program. I understand that. I don't have any argument with it. I am just trying to figure out how they came to that type of a cut for children's hospitals. You know, did you cut the program, was the program cut to lessen the part of that $99 million to any particular part of the country? You didn't do that.

MS. NESSELER. Sir, I think we are looking at putting the money to the highest priority needs, and there are other priority needs in the Federal government.

MR. HALL. What are those priority needs? Are you talking about low income areas?

MS. NESSELER. One could be the National Health Service Corps. Money is being put into the National Health Service Corps that provides money for pediatricians to go out to work in underserved areas in the United States.

MR. HALL. Working under what?

MS. NESSELER. The National Health Service Corps, sir. Or the Community Health Center program, which provides more community health services in local communities and rural communities. Those would be two programs I could cite as programs that are high priority needs for the President.

MR. HALL. You take unmet needs into consideration, you think, in arriving at that cut?

MS. NESSELER. Yes, sir.

MR. HALL. An unmet need's an unmet need, isn't it?

MS. NESSELER. Yes, sir.

MR. HALL. So, let us talk about that a little bit. Are you trying to funnel the money into the most needy areas? Is that what you are doing?

MS. NESSELER. Into the most priority areas--

MR. HALL. The most needy--

MS. NESSELER. Yes, sir. Not necessarily needy areas, but priority areas.

MR. HALL. How did you calculate that cut? Was it done on a percentage basis, a percentage of the needs, like some Medicaid areas would have a greater percentage of low income people?

MS. NESSELER. We are looking at the hospitals that can train the highest number of pediatricians or physicians, that can show the greatest financial need, and can show that they treat the largest number of uninsured. We are still under discussion on how those calculations will be made.

MR. HALL. Well, that would really not go to the rural areas. If it is for the largest number, it would go to the most densely populated areas, wouldn't it?

MS. NESSELER. Sir, we are looking at how we will make that calculation. That is under discussion.

MR. HALL. Who is looking at it? You have already done it. You have cut it from $299 million to $99 million, so nobody is looking, apparently. And this Congress is going to look at it.

MR. DEAL. The gentleman's time has expired.

MR. HALL. In that case, I will yield back my time.

MR. DEAL. I felt sure you would. Ms. Capps, you are recognized for your questions.

MS. CAPPS. Thank you, Mr. Chairman. I want to thank my colleague from Texas for setting this up, and acknowledging, Ms. Nesseler, that you are a maternal child health nurse--

MS. NESSELER. Yes.

MS. CAPPS. --and I am a public health nurse.

MS. NESSELER. Wonderful.

MS. CAPPS. I worked in my career with schoolchildren, and I don't know how anybody could say with a straight face that $99 million is an adequate amount for the Federal government to be putting into children's hospitals graduate medical education.

And I am also taken aback a bit with our Chairman's comment that there is a great deal of private money, and I am thinking of the families I know and you worked with, where the tragic situation of a serious, serious chronic health condition and no resources of any kind of private money, and these are the hospitals where our families go with our children. And I want to ask you about something particular to California and some other states.

MS. NESSELER. Yes, ma'am.

MS. CAPPS. The Administration's proposal would change the funding formula to place greater weight on the number of uninsured patients the hospital is treating. This kind of formula is not a factor in determining funding, though, for graduate medical education in adult hospitals, right?

MS. NESSELER. I am not an expert on GRM in adult hospitals.

MS. CAPPS. Okay. I am sorry. We--

MS. NESSELER. I am really not an expert on this but we could provide an answer for the record.

MS. CAPPS. California, among other states, is on the forefront, but not the only State, of expanding health coverage for more and more children. Surely, that is a commendable goal. Hopefully, we will be able, eventually, to have all children covered. Children's hospitals equally in California treat patients with or without health insurance. Funding for training programs affects the number of residents who can be trained. The changes to the funding formula the Administration is proposing would, in essence, punish children's hospitals in States that are making strides toward covering more children, even though the need to train more pediatric residents still exists, no matter how many of the patients are insured or uninsured.

However, without full funding, children's hospitals will have to cut their training programs, and still treat the same number of patients. How do you reconcile this, and why is there so much inequity when it comes to funding graduate medical education at children's hospitals?

MS. NESSELER. There is a limited source of Federal funding, and we are looking at putting our money into other high priority needs, ma'am.

MS. CAPPS. Higher priority needs than children's hospitals medical education?

MS. NESSELER. We are trying to direct healthcare services out to our populations, ma'am.

MS. CAPPS. Would you tell me anything that is a higher priority than that? You said direct medical service to patients.

MS. NESSELER. Through community health centers and the National Health Service Corps, where we are getting pediatricians out to the communities to provide direct healthcare services. There are two examples--

MS. CAPPS. But they are being trained at these hospitals with 66 percent less funding, or 67 percent less funding. Does that fit?

MS. NESSELER. The President believes that it is sufficient funding for children's hospitals graduate medical education, with the limited source of Federal funding that we have and our priorities. Yes, ma'am.

MS. CAPPS. Okay. Let me try something else, for 16 seconds. In your testimony--

MR. DEAL. That is over, not under.

MS. CAPPS. All right. I will wait. Thank you very much.

MR. DEAL. The gentlelady misunderstood the Chairman's question with regard to private funding. I was speaking of private funding for the hospitals themselves, not the families.

MS. CAPPS. I totally understand.

MR. DEAL. My hospitals are very well supported in my State with private funds that go along with the other funding sources. That was the point I was making.

MS. CAPPS. I guess I would beg to differ, that all States maybe aren't as blessed as yours.

MR. DEAL. Well, we set a good example in Georgia. I recognize Dr. Burgess for his questions.

MR. BURGESS. Thank you, Mr. Chairman. I apologize for being out of the committee hearing while we heard testimony.

Just for my basic knowledge, forgive me if this is ground that has already been covered. Mr. Chairman, do we just get three minutes for questions?

MR. DEAL. You didn't give your opening statement.

MR. BURGESS. Are there other sources of graduate medical education funding? The Chairman already referenced money that may be available in the community. Are there other sources for this funding, other than what is provided by the Federal government?

MS. NESSELER. From the Federal government for Children's Hospitals Graduate Medical Education, there is a small amount of Medicare dollars that goes to the children's hospital if they are treating chronic diseases. And State Medicaid dollars are a bit of a contribution also, in addition to some private funding dollars.

MR. BURGESS. Since, what do we see in our packet, 75 to 80 percent of the graduates who graduate from training programs in children's hospitals stay within a hundred mile radius of that hospital for their practice, is it appropriate for the communities that benefit from the training program, do in fact contribute? They are receiving something of value, which is a well trained pediatrician or pediatric sub-specialist in their community. Is it appropriate that we look to the private sector for some of that funding, as the Chairman has pointed out, that they do so well in Georgia.

MS. NESSELER. Sir, I can get an answer to that question for the record. I don't think I am prepared to discuss if private funding is fair to the communities.

MR. BURGESS. All right. I think I understand this, but just so that I get it for the record, is there a difference in the way that funding for graduate medical education primarily aimed at adult hospitals, is there a difference between that and the graduate medical education for children's hospitals?

MS. NESSELER. Again, I am not as familiar with the adult hospitals as I am with the children's hospitals graduate medical education program, and I don't feel--

MR. BURGESS. Do you think there is a monetary--to the amount that an adult hospital would receive, as opposed to a children's hospital?

MS. NESSELER. Well, a children's hospital is receiving money to help to adjust for the higher cost of care of severely ill children.

MR. BURGESS. As the program is currently run, do all hospitals who apply for graduate medical education receive that funding?

MS. NESSELER. Yes, sir. All 61 that apply receive funding.

MR. BURGESS. And then, is that allocation equal amongst the 61, or are there other factors that enter into that?

MS. NESSELER. There are other factors that enter into that, the direct medical education and indirect medical education. If you look at the number of residents, the FTE counts of number of residents, and you look at their case mix index, and the other factors I discussed.

MR. BURGESS. But you don't penalize the Chairman there in Georgia, because they get so much private funding. Let me ask you this. The gentlelady from California, they have done a wonderful thing in California with the Medical Injury Compensation Reform Act of 1975. We have done a good thing down in Texas with the so-called stacked cap that we passed in September 2003. Has liability reform in these States made a difference in the money available for children's hospitals? That would go off the expense side, I guess, rather than the near side, but I just can't help but feel that the money spent for providing for liability protection--

MS. NESSELER. I understand, yes.

MR. BURGESS. Is there any thought to providing any of the protection under the Federal Tort Claims Act for children's hospitals, especially those that are funded primarily from governmental sources?

MS. NESSELER. I believe not at this point.

MR. BURGESS. Mr. Chairman, I will yield back. You have been very indulgent.

MR. DEAL. I thank the gentleman. Mr. Pallone, you are recognized for questions.

MR. PALLONE. Thank you, Mr. Chairman.

I am getting a little upset here, from what I am hearing, and I don't mean to, in any way be upset with you, but the concern I have, as you know, when I did my opening statement, I talked about how I feel that there is discrimination in Federal programs against children. In other words, that when we do funding, or when we prioritize, seniors always seem to get the short end, and I am just concerned that what I am hearing now from the President's proposed changes here, simply aggravate that situation even more.

I mean, the way I see it, Ms. Nesseler, this program with the children's hospitals GME, was set up because there was a feeling that these children's hospitals weren't getting enough money, because they didn't have the Medicare patients, since they didn't have a large senior caseload through Medicare.

MS. NESSELER. That is correct.

MR. PALLONE. That we needed to do something to make up for it. Well, if you then say okay, this is not a priority for us any more, and we are just going to help those hospitals that are in crisis because they have a large number of uninsured or whatever, it just seems to me you are magnifying that problem that I am citing, in terms of a shortfall for children and children's hospitals, all the more. I mean, what are the Administration's priorities? I mean, would you advocate doing the same thing for adult hospitals? Would you say, okay, let us do this for adult hospitals. Let us just provide funding for crisis hospitals? I mean, how can they justify doing this for children's hospitals, knowing very well that this program was set up because of a disparity?

MS. NESSELER. That is correct. The program was for the disparity, and we do believe, though, that $99 million will help with that disparity gap, and we do believe that. The CMS funding for the adult hospitals, I don't have that program under my purview, so I can't comment on if I believe that should be cut or not, sir.

MR. PALLONE. So, what has been changed? In other words, what has changed? We know that this program was set up because of the disparity. You admit that the disparity existed. That is why we set up this--

MS. NESSELER. Yes, sir.

MR. PALLONE. What has changed? I don't see, I am sorry. I don't see the Administration proposing this for adult hospitals, so why has this situation changed now? I mean, what is your counterargument to the fact that--and essentially, I see this change as making the disparity even worse between children's hospitals and adult hospitals.

MS. NESSELER. Sir, we are targeting the limited amount of Federal dollars that there are, and we are targeting that to our hospitals with the greatest financial need that treat the most uncompensated care patients, to reach the best outcomes.

MR. PALLONE. But I mean, that is not happening with the adult hospitals that are linked to Medicare in their funding formula. So, wouldn't you have to conclude that this Administration is, again, aggravating this disparity for children?

MS. NESSELER. Sir, I don't run the CMS program. And I don't--

MR. PALLONE. Well, I mean, I can say from what I know--

MS. NESSELER. --know about adult healthcare.

MR. PALLONE. --that that is not happening with the adult hospitals. We don't have that similar type of proposal here in front of us. Our committee deals with adult hospitals. That is not the case. So, it just seems to me that this is just aggravating this disparity, making it worse, and making it easier to argue that this Administration is not concerned as much about children as they would be about adults. I mean, I don't know what else to say. I don't want to be so cruel, because I honestly feel that it is a problem that isn't just this Administration, but exists in general.

MR. BROWN. Would the gentleman yield?

MR. PALLONE. Yeah.

MR. BROWN. I hear you come back to that $99 million figure. The last two years, this Congress, bipartisanly, has appropriated, I believe $298 and $302 for these programs. Does that mean that these children's hospitals got overpaid $199 million, or $201 million, or whatever the numbers are, did we waste that money? Did Children's in Akron and Cleveland and Chicago and all over the country get too much money for graduate medical education, that they squandered? You keep coming back to that $99 million. You have never told us why it should be $99 million, other than the President says it should be $99 million. Was that money just something we wasted in this Congress, the extra $200 million the last two years?

MS. NESSELER. We are supportive of the Children's Hospitals Graduate Medical Education Program. We are supportive of children's care. We have a limited amount of Federal dollars, and we are putting those into our high priority areas, sir.

MR. PALLONE. Well, I mean, I understand. I just say that I think that what is happening here is increasing the disparity for children's care, and again, shows discrimination against children. I think that is clear. But I don't expect you to keep commenting on it, but that is my opinion.

Thank you.

MR. DEAL. I have had a unanimous consent request from Mr. Hall that he be allowed to ask an additional question, and I would extend that request to Ms. Capps, in the event she returns before we complete this witness. And without objection, it is allowed. Mr. Hall.

MR. HALL. Ms. Nesseler, I am sorry for you, to have to come over here. And you are doing a great job. You are carrying out your duties well, and I admire you for it. I just don't agree with the things that you are having to testify to. You talk about disparity. I live in the smallest county in Texas, geographically, and we are experiencing a children's population growth of about 8 percent. We are not experiencing any population growth of senior citizens or adults. They are dying off. They are going the other way.

I don't understand how, did you treat adult teaching hospitals any different than you treated children's teaching hospitals?

MS. NESSELER. Sir, I don't administer the adult hospitals, so I cannot comment on that.

MR. HALL. Would it surprise you that they were treated quite differently?

MS. NESSELER. I am not even sure if they were treated quite differently, sir.

MR. HALL. But it would or wouldn't surprise you if they were. You don't have to answer that. I don't think you are prepared to answer that one. I just wanted to get that into the record, about the disparity position, and the population growth going one way with children, and the other way with adults, and children getting this treatment. I can't believe that the adults got that treatment, this whole room would be full, and crowded out into the streets with adults here complaining about it. And we don't have that situation.

Mr. Chairman, thanks for letting me ask her that one question.

MR. DEAL. Ms. Capps, you are recognized for additional questions.

MS. CAPPS. I will pose this, but I have a feeling that it is not going to be answered, but I want to get it out anyway, Ms. Nesseler.

MS. NESSELER. Yes, ma'am.

MS. CAPPS. In your testimony, you stated that the President requests $99 million to support the mission of children's teaching hospitals. Children's hospitals already get 80 percent of the funding that other GME hospitals receive, so I imagine that percentage is going to be downsized a bit. But this amount is a great improvement over the percentage that children's hospitals received before children's GME was authorized, but it is still a discrepancy that is now going to be going in the wrong direction. We were hoping that we would be taking it closer to parity with adults.

Given this discrepancy, well, first of all, I guess I would like to ask you if there is a rationale for why we have a disparity between funding for children's medical education and adult, that somehow, it is of lesser, it is easier, or lesser value, I don't know, whatever you could answer to that. But given the discrepancy, I am wondering if you can give us some basis on which to justify the decision to cut the funding now by two thirds, and suggest that these funds would still support the mission of the children's teaching hospitals. In other words, why fund it at all, when we are going to be cutting so dramatically the amount that the Federal government has invested?

It is estimated that the cuts to children's GME funding would lead to tremendous financial losses on the part of the teaching hospitals. I mean for those that don't have enormous amounts of private funding, they are going to be looking at solvency, not even solvency, but being able to stay open and available.

And at the same time, we see the number of children losing private insurance coverage rising, and also, we have been asked in the very same budget to cut Medicaid reimbursement. So, it looks to me like we are pointing toward a perfect storm.

I am wondering, first of all, is there something within HRSA that gives a rationale for a disparity, percentage-wise, between funding for children's medical education and adult, and from however you could do it, and secondly, is there any awareness of what this could do to the presence of children's hospitals throughout the country?

MS. NESSELER. Ma'am, the first question, again, I have to state that the adult hospital program is run through CMS, not through HRSA, and I am not able to comment on that program.

MS. CAPPS. Well, let me ask is there conversation back and forth between the two?

MS. NESSELER. Yes, we have conversations with CMS regularly.

MS. CAPPS. You never brought this up with anybody?

MS. NESSELER. I have not personally, no. But we can get an answer for the record for you.

MS. CAPPS. I would really appreciate that.

MS. NESSELER. Yes, ma'am.

MS. CAPPS. I think it is important that we understand, I guess, the philosophy behind it, whether or not this is something that is intended, or is just because it has always been that way, or something like that.

But let me ask you, because you don't just talk to CMS, you must have some conservations with the teaching hospitals throughout the country, as you are determining your budget and your priorities.

MS. NESSELER. Yes, we do. We work closely with the children's hospitals, the 61 in the United States. We have a website. We do technical assistance, conference calls, we do technical assistance workshops, work closely with the children's hospitals--

MS. CAPPS. And we are going to hear from--

MS. NESSELER. Yes.

MS. CAPPS. --directly from them.

MS. NESSELER. Yes, ma'am.

MS. CAPPS. But I am wondering if you had gotten any feedback, and this isn't a surprise today, what has the reaction been to your office or to you, from some of the hospitals, in terms of what this is going to do to their funding source? Or their solvency, their ability to provide services, and to provide training?

MS. NESSELER. They understand that the Department has a priority list of programs that are a high priority, and they know that we have a good working relationship with them, and that we will all do the best that we can with our $99 million, and we believe we are supportive of the program with $99 million, ma'am.

MR. DEAL. Thank you, Ms. Nesseler. We appreciate your being here today, and some of the areas that you alluded that you would get further responses, we would encourage you to do that as soon as possible.

MS. NESSELER. Thank you, sir.

MR. DEAL. Thank you very much.

MS. NESSELER. I appreciate it.

MR. DEAL. Now, our second panel, if you would come to the table.

Welcome, gentlemen. We are pleased to have as our second panel, Mr. Patrick Magoon, who is President and CEO of the Children's Memorial Hospital in Chicago, Illinois; and Mr. Bill Considine, who is President and CEO of the Akron Children's Hospital in Akron, Ohio.

We are pleased to have both of you here. As I said earlier, your written testimony has been made a part of the record, and we would invite you to summarize in your opening statements.

Mr. Magoon.

STATEMENTS OF PATRICK MAGOON, PRESIDENT AND CEO, CHILDREN'S MEMORIAL HOSPITAL, CHICAGO, ILLINOIS; AND WILLIAM H. CONSIDINE, PRESIDENT AND CEO, AKRON CHILDREN'S HOSPITAL, AKRON, OHIO

MR. MAGOON. Thank you, sir. Mr. Chairman and subcommittee members, it truly is a privilege to be here with you this morning.

A few points about Children's Memorial Hospital. We happen to be the only full service children's hospital in the State of Illinois, and have the privilege of serving about 102,000 individual children who come to us from every county in the State of Illinois, from every area--urban, rural, and suburban. We happen to train about 92 pediatric residents, about 75 fellows, and about 100 medical students at our institution.

We are home to one of five independent, freestanding research centers which focus on providing research into the prevention and cures for diseases of children, and we also happen to be the single largest provider of pediatric Medicaid services in the State of Illinois, a State which does not provide Medicaid funding in support of the GME program.

I would like to make three points about the children's hospitals GME program. First, the goal of equity. Second, is its importance in terms of the training of the next generation of pediatricians and specialists for this country, and the importance of its investment in all children of our country.

First, as you know, CHGME's goal is to provide equitable Federal GME support to independent children's hospitals. Until GME financial reform is achieved, it is an interim step for our hospitals to receive Federal GME support comparable to what other teaching hospitals receive, and it enables us to make that multiyear commitment needed to train physicians.

Second, it has been a huge success in bolstering our ability to turn around a decline in the size of our training programs, and to strengthen them, at a time of a National pediatric workforce shortage.

Third, CHGME is an essential and yet critical investment in the future health of every child in the United States, because the Nation's 60 independent children's teaching hospitals are the backbone of healthcare for all.

But to start, I have to go back to the late 1990s. Healthcare price competition was intense. Children's hospitals faced enormous pressure because we do everything an academic medical center does, but with no Federal GME support, because we care for children, not the elderly. So why should that matter? In 1998, Medicare paid a teaching hospital, on average, more than $60,000 per full-time resident FTE, but paid an independent children's hospital less than $400. If there had been another major payer for GME, it really wouldn't have mattered, but private payers have stopped paying for the extra cost of teaching, and Medicaid payment for GME, as you know, is well below cost.

The lack of equitable Federal GME support put our hospitals truly at grave risk. By the late 1990s, children's hospitals nationwide began to face serious budget shortfalls. That, accompanied with the pressure mounting for the demand for services for children, really has created significant problems. In the case of the Children's Memorial Hospital, at that time, we were losing about $12.5 million on our operating performance at a very critical time. Our Medicaid losses totaled more than $23 million.

We took a very aggressive look at the operating performance for the institution. We reduced 400 positions, cut $25 million out of our operating budget, looked at every opportunity for efficiencies, but chose cognitively not to make a reduction in our training program because of its importance to our mission to train physicians, to improve research, and to really enable us to provide clinical care to our population.

In 1998 and in 1999, Children's Hospital went to Congress. We told our story. Few realized that independent children's teaching hospitals were basically left out in the cold when it came to Federal GME support. They clearly understood the issue of equity. Congress responded overwhelmingly with bipartisan support that led to CHGME's enactment in 1999 and reauthorization in 2000. We are deeply grateful to this subcommittee and the full committee for your leadership.

Today, children's hospitals GME provides, on average, about 80 percent of the Federal GME support other teaching hospitals receive through Medicare. It has made an enormous difference. Over the past five years, Children's Hospital has increased our training of pediatricians by 20 percent, and our pediatric specialists by 47 percent. Without this growth, the number of pediatricians would have continued to decline, and our training accounted for more than 60 percent of all new pediatric specialists, many who are in very, very short supply.

There is no better proof of CHGME's importance to all of pediatrics than the testimony of pediatric department chairs of medical schools. This spring, 80 pediatric department chairs asked the committee to continue CHGME. More than half have hospitals that receive no CHGME, but they know that independent children's hospitals are indispensable components of the training program. Why? Why did they take this position? We are only 1 percent of all of the hospitals in the Nation, but we train nearly 30 percent of all of the pediatricians, and half of the pediatric sub-specialists. We provide half of all specialty care for the sickest children, such as cancer, birth defects, and we are clearly the safety net to the poorest in our community.

In short, we are only one percent, but we do what touches children's lives each and every day. We train those pediatricians, we help with breakthroughs in medicine, and our researchers do everything they can to help discover the precursors to adult disease. That is why CHGME is an investment in the healthcare of all of our citizens. It is an investment in our teaching which translates into return on investment with respect to improved clinical care, research, and the ability to serve children.

We are grateful for the overwhelming support of the members of the House that they have provided for this program, and we respectfully ask that you continue this goal of equity, its success for expanding the pediatric workforce, and its investment in every child in our Nation.

Thank you very much, sir.

[The prepared statement of Patrick Magoon follows:]

PREPARED STATEMENT OF PATRICK MAGOON, PRESIDENT AND CEO, CHILDREN'S MEMORIAL HOSPITAL, CHICAGO, IL

MR. CHAIRMAN AND MEMBERS OF THE SUBCOMMITTEE, IT IS AN HONOR FOR ME TO BE HERE TODAY. I AM PATRICK MAGOON, PRESIDENT AND CEO OF CHILDREN'S MEMORIAL HOSPITAL IN CHICAGO, ILLINOIS. THANK YOU FOR THE OPPORTUNITY TO TESTIFY ON BEHALF OF THE FEDERAL CHILDREN'S HOSPITALS GRADUATE MEDICAL EDUCATION (CHGME) PROGRAM.

CHILDREN'S MEMORIAL WAS FOUNDED IN 1882 BY JULIA FOSTER PORTER WHO LOST HER SON TO ILLNESS. THE HOSPITAL BEGAN AS AN EIGHT BED COTTAGE AND HAS EVOLVED INTO A MAJOR MEDICAL CENTER THAT TODAY OWNS AND OPERATES 270 LICENSED BEDS AS WELL AS A FULL RANGE OF INPATIENT AND OUTPATIENT CARE AND RELATED ANCILLARY SERVICES. CHILDREN'S MEMORIAL IS ILLINOIS' ONLY INDEPENDENT, ACUTE CARE HOSPITAL DEDICATED EXCLUSIVLEY TO CHILDREN.

BECAUSE OF THE DEPTH AND BREADTH OF SERVICES WE OFFER, WE HAVE THE PRIVILEGE OF SERVING CHILDREN FROM EVERY COUNTY IN THE STATE. FOR EXAMPLE, FROM DURING FY 2002-2005, WE HAD 46,658 PATIENT ENCOUNTERS FROM CONGRESSMAN RUSH'S CONGRESSIONAL DISTRICT LOCATED ON THE SOUTH SIDE OF CHICAGO AND 384 PATIENT ENCOUNTERS WITH CHILDREN FROM CONGRESSMAN SHIMKUS' DISTRICT LOCATED DOWNSTATE.

OUR HOSPITAL TRAINS MORE DOCTORS FOR CHILDREN, PROVIDES MORE HOSPITAL CARE FOR CHILDREN, CONDUCTS MORE RESEARCH FOR CHILDREN, AND SERVES MORE MEDICAID PATIENTS THAN ANY OTHER HOSPITAL IN ILLINOIS. MEDICAID REPRESENTS 48% OF OUR INPATIENT CARE.

I WANT TO MAKE THREE POINTS ABOUT CHGME'S GOAL OF EQUITY, ITS SUCCESS FOR PEDIATRIC TRAINING, AND ITS INVESTMENT IN THE HEALTH OF ALL CHILDREN.

- FIRST, CHGME'S GOAL IS TO PROVIDE EQUITABLE FEDERAL GME SUPPORT TO INDEPENDENT CHILDREN'S HOSPITALS. UNTIL COMPREHENSIVE GME FINANCING REFORM IS ACHIEVED, CHGME IS AN INTERIM STEP FOR CHILDREN'S HOSPITALS TO RECEIVE NO MORE BUT NO LESS THAN THE FEDERAL GME SUPPORT THAT ALL OTHER TEACHING HOSPITALS HAVE RECEIVED FOR DECADES.
- SECOND, CHGME IS A SUCCESS IN BOOSTING OUR ABILITY TO BOTH TURN AROUND A DECLINE IN THE SIZE OF OUR TRAINING PROGRAMS AND STRENGTHEN THEM AT A TIME OF NATIONAL PEDIATRIC WORKFORCE SHORTAGES – WITHOUT HAVING TO SACRIFICE CLINICAL CARE OR RESEARCH.

- THIRD, CHGME IS AN INVESTMENT IN THE FUTURE HEALTH OF EVERY CHILD IN THE U.S. BECAUSE THE NATION'S 60 INDEPENDENT CHILDREN'S TEACHING HOSPITALS ARE THE BACKBONE OF HEALTH CARE FOR ALL CHILDREN.

BUT TO START, I HAVE TO GO BACK TO THE LATE 1990S. PRICE COMPETITION THEN, AS NOW, WAS INTENSE IN THE HEALTH CARE MARKETPLACE. INDEPENDENT CHILDREN'S HOSPITALS FACED ENORMOUS PRESSURES BECAUSE WE DO EVERYTING ANY ACADEMIC MEDICAL CENTER DOES – BUT WITH NO FEDERAL GME SUPPORT, BECAUSE WE CARED FOR VIRTUALLY NO MEDICARE PATIENTS.

WHY SHOULD THAT MATTER? IN 1998, MEDICARE PAID A TEACHING HOSPITAL, ON AVERAGE MORE THAN $60,000 PER FULL TIME EQUIVALENT RESIDENT, DIRECT AND INDIRECT MEDICAL EDUCATION FUNDING COMBINED. BUT, IT PAID AN INDEPENDENT CHILDREN'S HOSPITAL LESS THAN $400 PER RESIDENT.

IF THERE HAD BEEN OTHER MAJOR PAYERS OF GME FOR CHILDREN'S HOSPITALS, IT WOULD NOT HAVE MATTERED. BUT PRIVATE PAYERS STOPPED PAYING THE EXTRA COSTS OF TEACHING AND MEDICAID PAYMENT FOR GME IS WELL BELOW ITS COST. THE LACK OF EQUITABLE FEDERAL GME SUPPORT PUT OUR HOSPITALS AND ALL OF OUR MISSIONS – CLINICAL CARE, TEACHING, AND RESEARCH – AT GRAVE RISK.

IN 1999, RALPH MULLER WAS THE FORMER CEO OF THE UNIVERSITY OF CHILCAGO HOSPITALS, WHICH HAS A NON-INDEPENDENT CHILDREN'S HOSPITAL THAT RECEIVES MEDICARE GME. IN EXPLAINING HIS SUPPORT FOR CHGME, HE ONCE SAID: "I DON'T KNOW HOW CHILDREN'S MEMORIAL CAN OPERATE WITHOUT MEDICARE GME SUPPORT. OUR HOSPITAL COULD NOT."

BY THE LATE 1990S, CHILDREN'S HOSPITALS NATIONWIDE FACED BUDGET SHORTFALLS, PRESSURES TO EXPAND AND MOUNTING DEMAND FOR OUR SERVICES. CONSIDER MY OWN HOSPITAL. CHILDREN'S MEMORIAL HAD MASSIVE BUDGET LOSSES. IN FISCAL YEAR 1997, WE HAD A $12.5 MILLION OPERATING LOSS. CHILDREN'S MEMORIAL'S MEDICAID OUTPTIENT LOSSES AGAINST OUR COSTS AMOUNTED TO $23 MILLION.

EVERY PROGRAM WITHOUT VIABLE INCOME – INCLUDING GME – WAS UNDER INTENSE PRESSURE TO CUT BACK. WE MADE PAINFUL DECISIONS SUCH AS THE ELIMINATION OF 400 JOBS. WE STREAMLINED OUR OPERATIONS AND CUT ALMOST $25 MILLION IN COSTS. BUT IF WE CUT TRAINING, IT WOULD HAVE HAD SEISMIC RAMIFICATIONS FOR OUR CLINICAL OPERATIONS AND RESEARCH ENTERPRISE, WHICH ARE INTEGRATED WITH OUR ACADEMIC PROGRAM.

THE IMPORTANCE OF PEDIATRIC RESEARCH CANNOT BE UNDERESTIMATED. THE ENTERPRISE OF SCIENTIFIC DISCOVERY IN HEALTH CARE DEPENDS ON THE STRONG ACADEMIC PROGRAMS OF TEACHING HOSPITALS. BY COMBINING RESEARCH AND TEACHING IN A SINGLE CLINICAL SETTING, TEACHING HOSPITALS COMBINE THE TWO CRITICAL INGREDIENTS FOR SUCCESSFUL SCIENTIFIC DISCOVERY IN MEDICINE – SCIENTIFIC BREAKTHROUGHS AND RAPID TRANSLATIONS OF THEM INTO PATIENT CARE.

THE TEACHING ENVIRONMENT ATTRACTS THE ACADEMICIANS DEVOTED TO RESEARCH AND DRAWS THE VOLUME AND SPECTRUM OF CASES UPON WHICH CLINICAL RESEARCH RELIES. THE TEACHING ENVIRONMENT CREATES THE INTELLECTUAL ATMOSPHERE THAT TESTS

THE CONVENTIONAL WISDOM OF DAY-TO-DAY HEALTH CARE AND FOSTERS QUESTIONS THAT LEAD TO SCIENTIFIC BREAKTHROUGHS.

SIMPLY PUT, INDEPENDENT CHILDREN'S TEACHING HOSPITALS ARE PROOF OF THE IMPORTANCE OF ACADEMIC MEDICINE TO SCIENTIFIC DISCOVERY ESSENTIAL TO IMPROVING CHILDREN'S HEALTH CARE.

SCIENTIFIC ADVANCES OF CHILDREN'S TEACHING HOSPITALS HAVE HELPED CHILDREN SURVIVE ONCE FATAL DISEASES SUCH AS POLIO, TO GROW AND THRIVE WITH ONCE CRIPPLING DISABILITIES SUCH AS CEREBRAL PALSY, AND TO BECOME ECONOMICALLY SELF-SUPPORTING ADULTS WITH CONDITIONS SUCH AS JUVENILE DIABETES AND SPINA BIFIDA. THIS IS WHY OUR HOSPITALS ARE CONSISTENTLY AMONG THE LEADING RECIPIENTS OF NIH GRANTS FOR BIOMEDICAL RESEARCH.

CHGME FUNDING IS EXTREMELY IMPORTANT TO THE ABILITY OF CHILDREN'S TEACHING HOSPITALS, INCLUDING OURS, TO FULFILL OUR MISSION OF TRAINING THE NEXT GENERATION OF PHYSICIANS SPECIALIZED IN THE CARE OF CHILDREN, IN ADDITION TO THE MISSIONS OF CLINICAL CARE, RESEARCH AND ADVOCACY FOR CHILDREN. IF WE CRIPPLE OUR TRAINING PROGRAM, WE CRIPPLE OUR RESEARCH PROGRAM.

IN 1998 AND 1999, CHILDREN'S HOSPITALS WENT TO CONGRESS. WE TOLD OUR STORY. FEW REALIZED THAT INDEPENDENT CHILDREN'S TEACHING HOSPITALS WERE BASICALLY LEFT OUT IN THE COLD WHEN IT CAME TO FEDERAL GME SUPPORT.

CONGRESS RESPONDED OVERWHELMINGLY WITH BIPARTISAN SUPPORT THAT LED TO THE ENACTMENT OF CHGME IN 1999 AND ITS REAUTHORIZATION IN 2000.

WE ARE DEEPLY GRATEFUL TO THIS SUBCOMIMTTEE AND THE FULL COMMITTEE FOR THE LEADERSHIP YOU PROVIDED. TODAY, CHGME PROVIDES, ON AVERAGE, TO OUR HOSPITALS ABOUT 80% OF THE FEDERAL GME SUPPORT OTHER TEACHING HOSPITALS RECEIVE THROUGH MEDICARE. IT HAS MADE AN ENOMROUS DIFFERENCE FOR OUR HOSPITALS AND FOR OUR TRAINING PROGRAMS.

OVER THE PAST FIVE YEARS, INDEPENDENT CHILDREN'S TEACHING HOSPITALS HAVE INCREASED OUR TRAINING OF PEDIATRICIANS BY 20% AND OUR TRAINING OF PEDIATRIC SPECIALISTS BY 47%. WITHOUT THIS GROWTH THE NUMBER OF PEDIATRICIANS IN THIS COUNTRY WOULD HAVE CONTINUED THEIR DECLINE. OUR TRAINING ACCOUNTED FOR MORE THAN 60 PERCENT OF ALL NEW PEDIATRIC SPECIALISTS – SPECIALISTS SUCH AS GASTROENTEROLOGISTS THAT ARE IN SUCH SHORT SUPPLY IT CAN TAKE A YEAR OR MORE TO FILL VACANCIES.

CHILDREN'S MEMORIAL IS ONE OF THE MAJOR PEDIATRIC TEACHING HOSPITALS IN THE COUNTRY. WE ARE AFFILIATED WITH NORTHWESERN UNIVERSITY'S FEINBERG SCHOOL OF MEDICINE. OUR RESIDENCY PROGRAM IS CONSISTENTLY ONE OF THE MOST SOUGHT AFTER NATIONALLY. IN 2004-2005, FOR EXAMPLE, WE RECEIVED MORE THAN 820 APPLICATIONS FOR 31 OPENINGS.

BETWEEN 6 SPECIALTIES AND 26 SUBSPECIALTIES, EACH YEAR WE TRAIN ABOUT 185 PHYSICIANS, ALMOST HALF -- CURRENTLY 84 -- ARE PEDATRIC RESIDENTS. THE REMAINDER ARE FELLOWS IN SUCH AREAS AS INFECTIOUS DISEASE, NEONATALOGY, CARDIOLOGY AND OTHER PEDIATRIC SUBSPECIALTIES. MORE THAN 200 MEDICAL STUDENTS ROTATE THROUGH THE HOSPITAL FOR CLINICAL CLERKSHIPS. IN FY 2005, WE TRAINED 200 FULL-TIME EQUIVALENT RESIDENTS AT OUR

INSTITUTION. THIS REPRESENTS A GROWTH OF 27% (42.7 ADDITIONAL RESIDENTS) IN OUR TRAINING PROGRAM SINCE FY 2000.

THE CHGME PROGRAM HAS ALLOWED US TO IMPLEMENT CUTTING EDGE CLINICAL PROGRAMS. FOR EXAMPLE, WE HAVE DEVELOPED A SMALL BOWEL AND SHORT GUT TRANSPLANT PROGRAM. WE CANNOT OPERATE THESE TYPES OF INTENSIVE CLINICAL PROGRAMS WITHOUT OUR REISDENCY TRAINING PROGAM.

THERE IS NO BETTER PROOF OF CHGME'S IMPORTANCE TO THE NATION'S PEDIATRIC WORKFORCE THAN THE TESTIMONY OF PEDIATRIC DEPARTMENTS OF MEDICAL SCHOOLS, MOST OF WHICH DO NOT HAVE AN INDEPENDENT CHILDREN'S HOSPITAL. THIS SPRING, 80 PEDIATRIC CHAIRS ASKED THE COMMITTEE TO CONTINUE CHGME. MORE THAN HALF REPRESENT HOSPITALS THAT RECEIVE NO CHGME. THEY KNOW INDEPENDENT CHILDREN'S TEACHING HOSPITALS ARE INDISPENSABLE.

WHY? WE ARE ONLY 1% OF ALL HOSPITALS. BUT, WE TRAIN 30% OF ALL PEDIATRICIANS, HALF OF ALL PEDIATRIC SPECIALISTS, AND MOST PEDIATRIC RESEARCHERS. WE PROVIDE HALF OF ALL SPECIALTY CARE FOR THE SICKEST CHILDREN – WITH CANCER, BIRTH DEFECTS, TRAUMA. WE ARE THE SAFETY NET TO THE POOREST CHILDREN. WE HOUSE THE ENGINES OF PEDIATRIC RESEARCH.

IN SHORT, INDEPENDENT CHILDREN'S TEACHING HOSPITALS ARE ESSENTIAL TO HEALTH CARE FOR EVERY CHILD IN THIS COUNTRY. WE'RE ONLY 1% BUT WHAT WE DO TOUCHES EVERY CHILD'S LIFE – BY CARE WE GIVE, BY PHYSICIANS WE TRAIN, BY BREAKTHROUGHS IN HEALTH CARE OUR RESEARCH DISCOVERS.

THAT'S WHY CHGME IS AN INVESTMENT IN THE HEALTH OF ALL CHILDREN. IT IS AN INVESTMENT IN OUR TEACHING, WHICH TRANSLATES INTO AN INVESTMENT IN OUR CLINICAL CARE, OUR RESEARCH, AND OUR ABILITY TO SERVE ALL CHILDREN.

WE ARE GRATEFUL FOR THE OVERWHELMING SUPPORT THAT THE MEMBERS OF THE HOUSE HAVE PROVIDED FOR THE CHGME PROGORAM AND FOR THE SUPPORT THAT OUR COLLEAGUES IN THE PEDIATRIC AND HOSPITAL COMMUNITIES HAVE SHOWN, INCLUDING THE AMERCIAN ACADEMY OF PEDIATRICS, ASSOCIATION OF MEDICAL SCHOOL PEDIATRIC DEPARTMENT CHAIRS, ASSOCIATION OF AMERICAN MEDICAL COLLEGES, AND AMERICAN HOSPITAL ASSOCIATION.

WE RESPECTFULLY ASK YOU TO CONTINUE CHGME'S GOAL OF EQUITY, ITS SUCCESS FOR THE PEDIATRIC WORFORCE, AND ITS INVESTMENT IN THE HEALTH CARE OF EVERY CHILD AND EVERY GRANDCHILD. PLEASE REAUTHORIZE CHGME.

One Page Summary
Testimony of Patrick Magoon
Children's Memorial Hospital
May 9, 2006

I want to make three points about CHGME.

- First, CHGME's goal is to provide equitable federal GME support to independent children's hospitals. Until comprehensive GME financing reform is achieved, CHGME is an interim step for children's hospitals to receive no more but no less than the federal GME support that all other teaching hospitals have received for decades.

In 1998, the federal government provided independent children's hospitals with about 0.5% of the level of federal GME support that it provided to all other teaching hospitals through Medicare. Today, thanks to CHGME, it provides about 80%, and it makes it possible for us to make the multi-year commitment we need to train residents.

- Second, CHGME is a success in boosting our ability to both turn around a decline in the size of our training programs and strengthen them at a time of national pediatric workforce shortages – without having to sacrifice clinical care or research.

  Thanks to CHGME, independent children's hospitals have increased the number of pediatric residents we train by 20 percent and the number of pediatric specialty residents by more than 40%. Without the growth in our training, the total number of pediatric residents nationwide would have declined at a time of national shortages of pediatric specialists.

- Third, CHGME is an investment in the future health of every child in the U.S. because the nation's 60 independent children's teaching hospitals <u>are the backbone of health care for all children.</u>

  Through our clinical care, research, and training, children's hospitals touch the lives of all children. CHGME funding is fundamental to our ability to maintain and strengthen our training programs, which in turn are fundamental to our clinical and research missions.

Children's Memorial is a perfect illustration. In the 1990s, we were losing money, cutting staff, and facing pressures to curtail training. Today, thanks to CHGME, we gave been able to increase our training by more than 25%, implement cutting edge clinical programs, and undertake new research.

MR. DEAL. Thank you. Mr. Considine.

MR. CONSIDINE. Thank you, Mr. Chairman, and thank you, Mr. Brown, and to all the committee members. My name is Bill Considine, and I have had the privilege of serving as the President and Chief Executive Officer of Akron Children's Hospital for 27 years, and it has truly blessed my life. I really appreciate being here today, and being given the opportunity to share with you the importance of the CHGME program, not only on children's healthcare, but very definitely, on the children's hospitals of our country.

Akron Children's Hospital has been part of our community for 116 years, and during that time, has developed a very rich heritage and tradition. Last year alone, we served patients from all the 51 counties in the State of Ohio, 22 States, as well as other counties. In total, we saw 433,000 children through all our programs, and 210,000 of those children were served in our primary care offices in the rural areas of our region.

We believe that our promise is to treat every child as if that child was our own, and to make sure our doors stay open to all children, regardless of their ability to pay. We are the largest pediatric healthcare provider in our region, and have relationships with literally dozens of other adult hospitals. We know that it is our responsibility to be child advocates and to speak up in public policy arenas such as these on the needs of our children, and when you talk about medical education, it very definitely is a key priority here in our country, as well as our region.

When you talk about children's hospitals, too, and you look at the five components of our mission, which are family-centered patient care, training and education, research, community service, and child advocacy, you can see that training and education has been part of who we are for literally over a century.

The first medical resident in the city of Akron was a pediatric resident at Children's Hospital in the early 1900s, and the first nursing student in the city of Akron was a nursing student in 1905, at Akron Children's. We are one of the founders of the Northeastern Ohio University College of Medicine, very proud of that relationship, and we are the only pediatric provider there.

When we look at the issue of graduate medical education, I can assure you my 27 years has shown me the ups and downs of dealing with the vagaries relative to payment for medical education. When we talk about the medical education and the graduate medical education fund that has been put together for children's hospitals with our trustees, our medical staff, parents, and the community leaders that we are involved with, we discuss four items. One is equity. The whole premise of this program, back in 1999, was to bring equity to the responsibilities that children's hospitals have, as compared to the adult hospitals.

Our partners in the medical school, as Mr. Magoon has already pointed out, benefited from Medicare GME funding coming to them. In our town, they were receiving approximately $65,000 per resident with the Medicare GME program. Since we couldn't qualify for that, we were receiving under $400 per resident, and then, in 1999, with some of the other cutbacks to Medicaid in our State, that became a huge challenge for us to maintain our promise to our community to be involved in medical education. So, equity is what this program is about, and the CHGME money has brought us up to about $55,000 a resident, still not at that $65,000 level, but closer, and I think we have heard the figure 80 percent.

The other component of the program we talk about is need. There definitely is a need out there for the training of pediatricians and sub-specialists in medicine. Prior to this program, we had to curtail our training initiatives because of funding issues, and we were capping the number of residents we trained at about 50 a year. With the money that has come to us through this graduate medical education funding, we have been able to increase that to 87 full-time equivalents per year, and we also have 380 residents from adult hospitals rotating to us to get their pediatric experience. Consequently, we have been able to reduce a decline, or turn around a decline of 13 percent in young people going into the pediatric sub-specialties and residencies to where we have seen an 18 percent increase in that. That is good return on the investment.

The other need we have is to be a financially viable organization to bondholders and others that come to us for care, and prior to this money coming to us, we were facing a deficit on our margin. In 2005, our margin at our hospital was 0.4 percent. If this graduate medical education money would go away, we would have a negative margin, operating on a margin of 1.1 percent, and this has helped us stabilize that, and answer the tough questions that we need to answer about being a viable institution that serves those 433,000 children.

The other component we talk about with our trustees, is this program successful? And I would suggest, and respectfully to this group, it has been very successful. The numbers I have shared with you, in terms of what we have been able to do, in terms of training more and more residents, is really remarkable, and of the residents we train, 75 percent of them do stay in Ohio, and 50 percent of them go into primary care, pediatrics, and are placed in rural areas that really do need service directed to those children. Enormous success.

The other thing we talk about is value, and we are always looking for return on the investment, and again, I would respectfully say there has been enormous return on this investment. We have talked about the Medicare GME program, and know that last year, $8 billion was directed to 1,000 teaching hospitals to train residents and adult physicians. This CHGME program last year generated $300 million, not $300 billion, but $300 million, compared to $8 billion, and it went to the 61 hospitals, and we trained 5,000 residents. There is a good comparison there, and you can see the return on that $300 million is greater than that return on that $8 billion.

I hate to compare ourselves with the adult hospital, but what we are really trying to get to is a level playing field with our colleagues that have the same kind of mission statement that we do.

Thank you, Mr. Chairman, for the time. As you can see, I am passionate about this program.

[The prepared statement of Bill Considine follows:]

PREPARED STATEMENT OF BILL CONSIDINE, PRESIDENT AND CEO, AKRON CHILDREN'S HOSPITAL, AKRON, OH

Mr. Chairman, Congressman Brown, and members of the subcommittee, I am Bill Considine, president of Akron Children's Hospital for more than 25 years.

Thank you for the opportunity to testify on the federal Children's Hospitals Graduate Medical Education (CHGME) Program. Akron Children's is one of the six hospitals in Ohio and 60 nationwide that qualify for CHGME. We very much appreciate the leadership of the Energy and Commerce Committee and so many members of this Subcommittee in authorizing the program in 1999 and reauthorizing it for five years in 2000.

CHGME strives to give the nation's 60 independent children's teaching hospitals a level of federal GME support comparable to what all other teaching hospitals receive through Medicare. CHGME has been a success for the children of Akron, the children of Ohio, and the children in every state in the country. It has enabled our hospitals to sustain and strengthen our training programs, which are a vital part of our mission and the care we provide.

Akron Children's Hospital is a good illustration of the range of services an independent children's hospital provides.

We provide nearly 43,700 days of inpatient care, as well as 433,000 outpatient visits in the hospital and in 14 neighborhood clinics and other facilities throughout the region. They include 205,000 primary care visits, 108,000 specialty care visits, 62,000 emergency care visits, and other care visits. We serve children from 51 Ohio counties and 22 states each year. We devote 44% of our patient care to children under Medicaid and that proportion is only growing.

Akron Children's is a major center of excellence for children with cancer, heart defects and trauma. As a consequence, the severity of care our hospital provides is nearly 70% greater than it is for community hospitals nationwide. We also conduct research in areas such as cancer, heart defects, emergency care, neonatal care, emergency medicine, infectious disease, and more.

Akron Children's has a long-standing commitment to training physicians. In the 1920s, our hospital was the first of any hospital in Akron to train physicians. Today we play a unique role in physician training in our region. We are part of an academic medical enterprise that includes a medical school with three university affiliations and eight teaching hospitals. Akron Children's is the only major pediatric institution.

In addition to training more than 70 pediatric and pediatric specialty residents annually, our hospital provides training to more than 380 residents in other areas – such as internists, family practice physicians, surgeons. They rotate from the other teaching hospitals through our hospital for short periods of time to receive exposure to pediatrics.

More than 75% of all of the pediatricians and pediatric specialists we train go on to practice in Ohio. More than half of the pediatricians we train provide care as part of our community based primary care network after graduation. And most of the pediatric subspecialists in our community are trained at the hospital. Our training program benefits not only our patients but all children.

In the late 1990s and early years of this decade, as CHGME was just starting, Akron Children's had major financial challenges. We faced negative operating margins, pressures to curtail our training, and pressures to curtail services for which little or no income was available. One example was our regional poison control, which we had to close for lack of funds. Another example was the closure of our "continuity" clinic which moved patients from the hospital to primary care clinics in the community.

While our adult teaching partners received more than $60,000 of dollars in Medicare GME support per resident, we received only a few hundred dollars per resident, with no comparable, alternative source of GME support. We were dedicated to our historic mission of physician education in our region, but it was becoming harder and harder to continue to shoulder our responsibility for training about 50 FTE residents at that time, much less strengthen that commitment to meet growing need.

Today, the $4 million in annual CHGME funding that Akron Children's receives has made a world of difference. We have increased the total number of FTE residents we train by 21%, the number pediatric FTE residents we train by 20%, and the number of pediatric specialists we train by much more since 2000. This year, we will train more than 87 FTE residents, including 71 pediatric residents and fellows with specialty programs in clinical areas such as emergency care, radiology, pathology, and sports medicine.

We have opened new training programs in pediatric oncology, pediatric palliative care, and child psychiatry. We are applying for approval to open programs in pediatric general surgery and burn care. Those new programs and the residents we train will help us to respond to serious physician shortages. For example, mental health care for children has been in a crisis in our region for many years. In the face of overwhelming need, Akron Children's itself was forced to scale back its inpatient psychiatric service. Thanks to CHGME funding, we are now able to train pediatric psychiatrists with a good chance they will practice in our region. That will help us to develop new services and meet the tremendous unmet need that exists.

We have been able to improve the quality of the training we provide in a number of ways. By employing hospitalists – full time, senior physicians on staff in the hospital -- we enhance the training experience of the residents. By being able to increase the physicians we employ, it makes it possible for faculty to devote more time to research, which enriches the research experience of our residents. Research is a growing part of our hospital's mission, and future pediatric researchers come primarily from independent children's hospitals.

With the resources CHGME has given us, we have been able to introduce new electronic technology – hand-held computers to aid residents in treating complex patients. We have expanded training to include new areas of focus on special dimensions of pediatric care, such as palliative care, which is so important with the growing numbers of children with cancer we treat.

And we have been able to do all of this without sacrificing our clinical care or research efforts. In fact, with CHGME, we have been able to strengthen both, as CHGME helped offset losses from the uncovered costs of teaching.

If there were no CHGME funding tomorrow, Akron Children's would find its operating margins in the red and its financial health at risk. Our ability to open new fellowships in surgery and burn care, which have been recommended by the American College of Surgeons, as well as our ability to continue to provide pediatric rotational training to hundreds of non-pediatric physicians would be in jeopardy. And our loss of nearly $4 million would, once again, put pressure to cut back on vital services for which there is little or no income, such as the physicians we now pay for to deliver care to low-income children at a community health center.

Our experience is reflected among the 60 independent children's hospitals. In the late 1990s, many faced financial challenges, which Moody's Investor Services and Standard and Poor's attributed in part to the absence of public funding for our education programs. Many of our hospitals had begun to curtail our training, limit services that require hospital subsidy or not undertake needed service expansions.

Since CHGME's enactment in 1999 and full funding for the first time in 2002, the picture has changed significantly. Collectively, we have increased the numbers of pediatric residents trained, the numbers of pediatric specialists trained, and the numbers, and the number of pediatric subspecialty training programs. Without our growth in training due to CHGME, the number of pediatric residents trained would have continued to decline.

Equitable GME support through CHGME helped offset our losses on teaching and that has helped us weather many challenges -- children's growing loss of private insurance, rising numbers of children covered by Medicaid for which payment is well below cost, mounting costs for information technology, and the ongoing capital needs of resource and service intensive institutions like ours.

In conclusion, CHGME restores equitable federal GME support and fair competition to children's hospitals. CHGME benefits all children.

There is strong, bipartisan support for CHGME. Please continue the strong, successful CHGME program that exists today by reauthorizing it as quickly as possible.

One Page Summary

Testimony by WilliamConsidine
Akron Children's Hospital

I. Greetings

II. Appreciation for the broad, bipartisan support for enactment and reauthorization of CHGME from Congress overall and the leadership of full committee and subcommittee.
- Authorization in 1999
- Reauthorization for five years in 2000

III. Akron Children's Hospital's commitment to training pediatric and specialty residents is historic.
- The first teaching hospital in Akron
- The single, major children's teaching hospital in our region, caring for children from 50 counties in Ohio and 22 states
- Today, train more than 80 FTE residents, including pediatric residents and other residents receiving pediatric rotations

IV. History of CHGME
- Began in the late 1990's when Akron Children's faced financial shortfalls: pressure to close poison control center, continuity clinic; ability to train only 50 residents with pressure to cut

V. Financial impact of CHGME on Akron Children's
- Offset the financial burden of training residents
- Increased pediatric resident trained by 20%
- Employment of new specialty physicians
- Introduction of electronic technology

VI. A future without CHGME
- Financial losses
- Curtailment of training
- Limiting services

VII. A request for reauthorization of GME funding

MR. DEAL. Well, thank you. Both of you made a very compelling testimony for us in this consideration, and I would be remiss if I didn't say thank you to both of you, and to you your institutions, for what you do to train pediatricians and those in pediatric specialties. As a grandfather, I am perhaps a little more acutely aware of children's healthcare, maybe, than I was when I was a father, but grandchildren seem to get your attention a little bit more sometimes.

You have heard the comments with regard to what the proposal is in the budget, to go to more of a needs basis assessment of allocation of funding. How would each of you think your institution would fare using that as almost the exclusive criteria? Mr. Magoon, I will start with you.

MR. MAGOON. Thank you, sir. I would suggest if one were to look at the industry, that is the children's hospitals, the 61 of us that are there, a change of this magnitude would reduce, on average, operating margins by about 33 percent. Prior to the program, the operating margins were somewhere in the range of a negative 4 percent to about 1, 1.5, so it would take many of our institutions, and put them in financial peril immediately. And that really works against our objective of having strong children's hospitals serve as the backbone of the healthcare system for our community, and really, they are the safety net provider. So, it puts our most vulnerable at risk, quite frankly, for immediate care.

In the long run, I would also say that we make a commitment to a resident for three years, and so, when you are done with that three year commitment, that resident goes off, but there is another resident right behind him, and behind her, and behind me. And what we also need to recognize is many of them go into sub-specialty areas of pediatric medicine, and I would just like to highlight two facts.

We have a fellowship program in pediatric orthopedic surgery, and we have not been able to fill that for the last 3 years. This year, there will be five individuals finishing their fellowship training in pediatric orthopedic surgery nationwide, to meet the needs nationwide. The other example I would share with you is pediatric endocrinology. Last year, there were eight individuals across the country who finished their fellowship training in pediatric endocrinology.

Contrast that to the challenge of obesity in America, the expansion of endocrine problems, and the fact that there are eight positions across the country, and it is no small wonder why there are long waits to see pediatric specialists across the Nation. You know, the challenge is significant.

MR. DEAL. Now, Mr. Considine, how would this kind of criteria affect your institution?

MR. CONSIDINE. Well, one of the questions I know that we would have to deal with at our trustee level is why was there a change in the premise of the initial program? When this program was put in place in 1999, it was to bring equity to children's hospitals that were involved in training at the graduate medical educational level, and bring that equity up to what the adult hospitals are.

And with this proposal, I see us now being pitted against our fellow children's hospitals, and having to make choices, which ones are more involved in serving the children of their region versus others. The amount of money that is still not there, to bring us up to that equity level. If there was a cutback at our place, as Mr. Magoon was pointing out, areas where we have been able to advance our fellowship training with these funds, we have been able to start fellowship trainings in palliative care, sports medicine, endocrinology, radiology, and we have been just approved for a fellowship in pediatric oncology, and also in pediatric psychiatry. And the American College of Surgeons has asked us to bring on board a fellowship in pediatric surgery and also burn care.

All of those areas are shortage areas, in terms of men and women choosing those as their professions, and if we were receiving a cutback, Mr. Chairman, we would have to think twice about whether or not we could bring those programs online.

MR. DEAL. Mr. Magoon, I believe you mentioned that your State did not provide State-funded medical education dollars. Is that what you said?

MR. MAGOON. Yes, sir.

MR. DEAL. What about Ohio, Mr. Considine?

MR. CONSIDINE. One of the challenges we had in 1999 is Ohio was moving to mandatory Medicaid managed care, and as they did that, the patients who went into the Medicaid managed care organizations, the dollars that used to follow them to us when they were through the State program, for medical education, those dollars disappeared. And the current program in Ohio is moving more and more statewide to Medicaid managed care, and the amount of money that we would receive through Medicaid for GME will dry up. It has been reduced substantially. Rainbow Babies and ourselves in Northeastern Ohio have been in counties that have been mandatory, so for example, all the patients that are Medicaid patients for our county, Summit County, we have received no GME money through Medicaid for them.

MR. DEAL. Thank you. Mr. Brown.

MR. BROWN. Thank you, Mr. Chairman. Mr. Magoon, thank you for your comments. They were particularly illuminating about pediatric endocrinology. I spoke just a few days ago with a pediatric specialist in endocrinology in Miami. You know, we talked about the higher rate of diabetes and obesity, and just what you spoke about, and I think that really underscores the importance of all of this.

Mr. Considine, talk for a moment, if you would, about other sources of GME funding for Akron Children's.

MR. CONSIDINE. Well, our main source right now is the children's hospitals GME program that we were talking about. There are funds, and they are dwindling, that come to us through the Medicaid program, and--

MR. BROWN. Could you sort of give us rough ballpark figures? You said you are up to $60,000, or up to $55,000 overall, so can you break down roughly how much of it is GME, how much of it is burn unit? Is there a way of doing that, roughly?

MR. CONSIDINE. Well, our burn unit also cares for adults, as you know. We are a regional burn center that cares for adults as well as kids. There are two children's hospitals in the country that do that, Arkansas Children's and ourselves. And Congressman, I--

MR. BROWN. Okay.

MR. CONSIDINE. --don't have that on the tip of my tongue, but there is a breakout there, and we do get a little more funding because of that to us, because of the adult component of that care.

MR. BROWN. And you get other funding, Medicaid and in-State if there are any significant dollars there?

MR. CONSIDINE. Not significant dollars, sir.

MR. BROWN. Okay. What are your thoughts on the previous witness', the Administration's proposal to target funding to, I believe, as Mr. Hall and she were going back and forth, to the neediest hospitals? What does that mean to Akron and to many hospitals, many of the freestanding children's hospitals?

MR. CONSIDINE. Well, during my 27 years, I have had the privilege of visiting a lot of our children's hospitals in this country, and the children that are served by those hospitals, they deserve the very best in terms of the care. There are needs for sub-specialists and primary care pediatricians in all the areas that are represented by those 61 children's hospitals, and I don't know how we could go through a process to determine which of those children's hospitals, and which children served by those hospitals are more needy than other children.

MR. BROWN. And $99 million just doesn't get there.

MR. CONSIDINE. Well, if we are not quite at the equity level with $300 million, you can run the math, $99 million would bring us down. It wouldn't bring us closer to equity with out adult counterparts.

MR. BROWN. Tell us about, you have mentioned that Akron General serves, I believe you said 50plus counties.

MR. CONSIDINE. Akron Children's.

MR. BROWN. I mean Akron Children's, I am sorry--50 plus counties. And that you are in an urban area, generally, you people, that Cleveland, Akron, that is a pretty populous area of the State, but obviously, you reach way beyond into Southeast Ohio, Eastern Ohio areas that are less populous. Tell us about the rural GME program, what that means in those communities, 50 miles, 75 miles, 100 miles south or west of Akron.

MR. CONSIDINE. Well, as you know, Congressman, we serve the largest Amish population, at the Children's Hospital, in the country, and we have established some primary care offices in the counties where the Amish reside, and those 14 office sites that I was speaking to, that are primary care office sites, that saw this 210,000 children right now, are offices that are based outside of Summit County. And one of the things the graduate medical education funding has helped us do is make sure that we have increased the number of residents so we can extend resident education into those offices in those counties. So, that definitely does enhance not only the training program that those residents are in, but the services being provided to the children of the folks that live in those communities.

MR. BROWN. Thank you, Mr. Chairman. Thank you.

MR. DEAL. Thank you. Mr. Hall, you are recognized for questions.

MR. HALL. I thank you, Mr. Chairman. I note that both of you are Presidents and CEOs, so you know what you are doing, and I referred to my own home county a moment ago, with the lady from the Administration, and I noted also that our children's population is growing ten times the national average there, and I hate to think about how far we would be behind if we didn't have this program. So, Mr. Considine, you are from Ohio, right?

MR. CONSIDINE. Yes, sir.

MR. HALL. Is that a similar situation in Ohio? You have that type dramatic growth in your area?

MR. CONSIDINE. We have some of our services that are seeing growth, but we have other components of our service area, quite honestly, that are not seeing that kind of growth. We are not as robust in population growth as your area, and that is one of the challenges of making sure we get a balance, in terms of the coverage in all those areas. But at no time, having children that aren't able to access the kind of care we would want for our children.

MR. HALL. I think they must have calculated their figures on what were needy areas. I think they must have tied it, probably, to Medicaid, and then done it on a percentage basis, which could mean, there is a little town in my county that is the fourth fastest growing city in the United States, and it is growing about 100 or 150 people a month, because they didn't start with much. But still, that statistic is there, and that could be part of what they based that on. Do you know she couldn't answer for us, the lady I was sorry for her, being that had to send her over here today. I would have hated to have been her. But do you know, what is the difference in adult teaching hospitals, the way they are treated with this budget than the children's teaching hospitals? Do you have that information?

MR. MAGOON. It is my understanding that there is no change in the Medicare program reimbursing the adult institutions, the change is specifically to this program, and to this population of institutions.

MR. HALL. Okay. Does direct medical education funding, when it is doled out on a per resident basis, a head count basis, does that adequately cover the cost to train an individual physician?

MR. CONSIDINE. No, sir, not in our case, and--

MR. HALL. How close does it come?

MR. CONSIDINE. Well, with the program we are talking about here, it has brought us to a more equitable level with our adult counterparts. We are about 80 percent of that. And we have discussions, too, about what we can include in the Medicare cost report as allowable costs. Some of the services that we extend with residents, out to our rural primary care clinics, for example, oftentimes some of those expenses cannot be included in those formulas.

Having said that, I think we are getting closer to equity because of the children's hospital GME Program, and that is why we are concerned about any cut in that program.

MR. HALL. Mr. Magoon.

MR. MAGOON. From an accountability point of view, we are required to report back in a very similar fashion to our adult counterparts on the effective use of those dollars. It is not without accountability. It is the very same accountability, in fact, we are required to go through any other fiscal intermediary on an annual basis, because the appropriation is annual. So, if anything, there is greater scrutiny and review of the appropriateness of the use of these funds in these 61 children's hospitals than across the country in general.

MR. HALL. Well, I really thank you two for taking the time from a very busy job to come here, and then to give us this testimony, and we have a Chairman that is probably one of the best subcommittee Chairman in this Congress, and I believe he is going to correct some of the Administration's problems on this. I am going to rely on him, too, and I am going to brag on him until he does.

I yield back my time.

MR. DEAL. You get a lot of things if you give him extra time for questions, you know.

Dr. Burgess, you are recognized for questions.

MR. BURGESS. Thank you, Mr. Chairman. I also want to thank our two witnesses for taking time out of their schedules and from their work to be here with us. I also want to acknowledge that there is with us in the audience a representative from a hospital down in Mr. Hall's and my neck of the woods, the Children's Medical Center of Dallas, and Maisy

James is with us today, and we appreciate her being here in the committee.

Mr. Hall correctly pointed out that the Administration's request for this year is far below what we should see in the final appropriations bill, but what was the first year, under this additional funding, what was the first year that the children's hospitals received additional funding under the children's graduate medical education?

MR. CONSIDINE. My recollection, it was maybe in 1999 or the year 2000, and I think the amount was $40 million, at a national basis.

MR. BURGESS. Yeah, in fiscal year '01, according to the figures I have, it was $235 million, a significant increase the next year, fiscal year 2002, was $285 million. Fiscal year '03, $290 million, fiscal year 2004, my first year here, was $303 million. It did decline a little bit after that, '05 was $301 million, and '06, with the across the board 1 percent cut that we did, was $297 million. So, although as Mr. Hall correctly pointed out, I wouldn't have wanted to be here arguing the Administration's position, I think we can see that the funding has been there, and it is incumbent upon us to make certain that that level stays.

I also feel obligated to point out for the committee that this is important work that these gentlemen do, and the pediatric specialists or the pediatric sub-specialist--children are not just little adults. They require a special expertise and a special gift to be able to provide the highly specialized care that children need. A surgeon who is trained in adult surgery cannot just overnight become a children's surgeon. It requires special training and special expertise, the management of fluids, everything about their medical care is considerably different, and it does require the application, the education of specialists.

One question I do have is has this funding allowed you to increase the number of medical residents that you educate?

MR. CONSIDINE. In our case, sir, it has dramatically assisted us in increasing the number of residents. In 1999, it was 50. Last year, it was 87 a year, and through our program, and it has also helped us bring fellowships online, and one of the other results of that is more patient activity is coming in through our doors, because of the increase of available manpower.

MR. BURGESS. Now, were children's hospitals affected in the year 2000, 2001, I don't remember which it was, when across the country, facilities that provided graduate medical education were required to adhere that resident's work hours be no more than 80 hours per week?

MR. CONSIDINE. Yes.

MR. BURGESS. So you all follow to those guidelines?

MR. CONSIDINE. Yes.

MR. BURGESS. Did that result in any requirement for increasing the number of residents that you retain?

MR. CONSIDINE. I think that is a critical factor driving--

MR. BURGESS. Because I remember they used to get 160 hours of work a week out of us at Parkland Hospital.

MR. MAGOON. Things have changed.

MR. CONSIDINE. It has, in fact, increased the demand for residents, and I think it has also improved the quality of education. Now, we have gone from roughly 62 to over 90 residents, because the funding is there, the patient demand is there. It is critically important, in terms of patient safety, and in particular, to meet the requirements for the 8 and 80 work rules.

MR. BURGESS. Now, the comment was made that private insurance no longer paid for education for graduate medical education children's hospitals, but they still reimburse you, you still get private insurance reimbursement for children who are covered, who have insurance coverage, correct?

MR. MAGOON. Yes, we do. In negotiations with commercial payers, they make it very clear that that is one of the areas they don't want to see loaded in their pricing.

MR. BURGESS. But that would be true for hospitals that train residents who practice adult medicine as well.

MR. MAGOON. Yes.

MR. BURGESS. So, that is across the board.

MR. MAGOON. That is across the board negotiation we get involved in.

MR. BURGESS. I do have to ask the question. I asked it of the HRSA person, and it probably was inappropriate for me to ask, but what have you noticed, has either of your States one of the States that has undergone a significant change in medical liability with passage of caps or any commitment to non-economic damages?

MR. MAGOON. Let me, if I may, relate one story. In the State of Illinois, there virtually is no professional liability insurance, quite frankly, in Cook County, Illinois. Our attachment point for our self-insurance program is $15 million. Consider that your deductible on your automobile insurance is $15 million. And there is no aggregate cap, so you can have as many $15 million in claims over the course of the year as they may arise. There is no aggregate cap, so in our particular circumstance, there virtually is no insurance, and while we buy about $80 million of excess coverage, predominantly offshore, you rarely ever penetrate any one of those layers. So, it is a huge issue for us, and while cap professional liability reform was passed last year, it still needs to be tested at the State Supreme Court level before we ever see any relief with respect to the insurance coverage. So, it is a huge burden for places like ours.

MR. BURGESS. I would just point out that in Texas, where we passed a constitutional amendment to allow that to happen, our not-for-profit hospitals, I think, have seen a significant benefit from having an aggregate cap on liability, and the hospitals were actually, it was an unintended consequence but a good consequence, that they received the benefit from that.

Mr. Chairman, I hope we will see some additional activity on that this year. With that, you have been very indulgent, and I will yield back.

MR. DEAL. Well, thank you. And gentlemen, thank you again for your presence and your testimony. It was excellent, and with that, this hearing is adjourned.

[Whereupon, at 4:35 p.m., the subcommittee was adjourned.]

APEX
TP
9780160770128
76901953 – 88